Stealing the Dragon's Fire

"I would recommend this book to women who are confronted with breast cancer, particularly those who have never had any serious illness before. It gave me a look at breast cancer from a patient's point of view to remind me of continued need for compassion and careful bedside manners."

Dr. Thomas S. Dawson, D.O., family physician
Bothell, Washington

"A much-needed resource manual and narrative for anyone suffering and surviving the trauma of cancer or terminal illness. Herein lies a formula for life."

Taylor Danard, M.A., psychotherapist
Seattle, Washington

"Clo manages to touch on every emotion I felt going through breast cancer. It is a 'must read' for anyone going through this ordeal, as well as families, friends, and those in the medical profession. It will give anyone reading it hope and courage."

Priscilla McCarty, breast cancer survivor
Bothell, Washington

"*Stealing the Dragon's Fire* was a Godsend to me. Only a few months after reading the manuscript, I received the news that my mother had breast cancer. As we began this frightening experience together, it was *not* a journey into the unknown; thanks to your book, I was prepared for all that happened and was able to support my mom and understand her needs. My mother had a mastectomy, six months of chemotherapy, and is now having a five-year follow-up series of tamoxifin. Mom's doctors credited her excellent attitude and her support system for her minimum of side effects. I credit your book for helping me support her on this challenging journey."

Norma L. Plumb, educator
Lynnwood, Washington

"The inspiring, moving account of Clo Wilson-Hashiguchi's journey through her mastectomy and recovery is essential reading for any person dealing with the complexities of cancer, either personally or with someone dear to them. She includes every aspect of emotion, both raw and humorous. It is essential to keep a box of tissues nearby while reading this book."

Eleanor L. (Ellie) Lange, family of cancer patient
Bothell, Washington

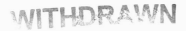

Stealing
the Dragon's Fire

A Personal Guide and Handbook
for Dealing with Breast Cancer

Clo Wilson-Hashiguchi

Illustrations by Monica Kumiko Hashiguchi
Photographs by Annette Porter
Technical Assistance by Brian Glenn Hashiguchi

Wilson Publishing
Bothell, Washington

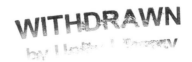

Published by
Wilson Publishing
P. O. Box 12634
Bothell, WA 98082-2634

7/01

Library of Congress Catalog 93-94147
ISBN 0-9638590-0-5

Dedication

To every person who must enter the lair of this
Dragon.

In memory of:
Penny Schick, Marie Baker, Marie McClintock, Tara
Havemeyer and all others who have lost their lives in
this battle.

I think over again my small adventures,
My fears
Those small ones that seemed so big
For all the vital things I had to get and to reach
And yet there is only one great thing
The only thing,
To live to see the great day that dawns,
And the light that fills the world.
                                    — Inuit Song

Acknowledgments

To Frank and Kay Wilson, my mother and father, who showed by their example that good health and quality of life are worth fighting for.

To Ralph Johnson, who believed in my worth, and supported that belief in many significant ways.

Mitzie Hashiguchi, who watched over me and my family with great care as I recovered from surgery, allowing me time to heal, as well as to keep a journal which supported the beginning of this book.

Brian and Monica, my courageous children, who braved this journey with me: To Brian, the first keen listener of the manuscript at nine years old, for being so willing to keep the computer going at all times of the night and day, and for putting together the bibliography, plus reviewing copy. To Monica, for carefully reviewing the manuscript, for sharing her image of the dragon of breast cancer in our home as a 10-year-old girl, (shown at the beginning of each chapter), and agreeing to use her artistic talent to be an outstanding illustrator of this book.

Glenn (Gooch), who kept the financial piece going, who did extra duty as a husband while I was recovering, and who encouraged me times when I might have given up.

Rob Roy, my brother, and his wife, Carol, for their strong support. To Judy, my sister, and her daughter, Connie, for their supportive belief in the project. To Jill, my sister-in-law who helped me believe I could survive.

Ellie Lange, who walked beside me daily giving me courage, not faltering throughout the long months and years, a steady guide through the dark places.

To Pat Feltin and Georgia Fawcett, great friends, and living evidence that women can survive breast cancer well.

To Issen Powter, who chose to hear my screams in the dark with love and great humor, and who helped me ready Stephen Meredith's transcript.

To my dear family and many wonderful friends, too numerous to mention, who extended themselves and their resources to be there in a loving way for us.

To Venice Maling, breast cancer survivor, whose courage inspired me in dealing with the disease and treatment as she traveled north to Alaska with her physician husband: a new home, a new medical practice, a new, life-threatening challenge, and chemotherapy treatments. I thought of her with compassion as I wrote this book.

To Annette Porter, breast cancer survivor, for choosing to support this project as an extraordinary photographer and friend, generously offering numerous hours and much insight into helping this project come together in the best possible way.

To Marie Baker, a dear and courageous human being, who shared her journey of breast cancer in many ways, including a personal interview.

To Bill Baker, who generously reviewed copy; Dr. Marleen Wekell, who made available to me many significant research articles regarding breast cancer; and Kelli Wilson, who helped put together two parts of the resource section.

To my extraordinary team of doctors:

Dr. Thomas S. Dawson, D.O., Family Physician, who supported me and my children with humor and sensitivity as I worked hard to recover, and who offered his time and energy to encourage me on my way with this book.

Dr. David Asmussen, Ob/Gyn, who first insisted I get a mammogram, then encouraged me and the emergence of this book with his suggestions and insight, and who first saw its possibilities as a handbook for women.

Dr. Stan Lennard, General Surgeon, who performed the mastectomy but, more than that, offered his kind support from one human being to another, who gave his continued support, valuable time, effort, and ideas to the emergence of this project.

Dr. Mukund Sargur, Oncologist, Hematologist, Internist, who monitored my adjuvant hormone therapy, and who continues to monitor my recovery from this disease, who believed in this book while it was yet a seed, and who supported my efforts with an extraordinary amount of time and energy with regard to the issues surrounding breast cancer.

To Dr. Eric Taylor, Radiation Oncologist, Evergreen Hospital(Kirkland, WA), for allowing me to view a patient going through radiation simulation, and radiation therapy in the radiation oncology department, in addition to granting me a personal interview, patiently answering my numerous questions regarding this treatment.

To Dr. Thomas Johnson, Radiation Oncologist, Group Health Hospital(Seattle WA), for allowing me to view and photograph a patient going through radiation treatments at the radiation oncology department, in addition to granting me a personal interview, and allowing Kevin Belcher, Radiation Technician, to also answer my many questions regarding radiation treatment.

To Group Health Hospital Oncology Department (Seattle, WA) for allowing us to photograph a patient going through chemotherapy treatments.

To Judith H.M. Jones, B.S., Cancer Information Specialist at Wellness Works, Evergreen Cancer Center, Evergreen Hospital, my heart-felt appreciation for the extensive support offered in multitudinal ways to make this book one that is valuable to all those who are touched by breast cancer. She increased the vision of this book by her continued willingness to share her knowledge and time.

To Sandra Johnson, M.S.W. Supervisor, Evergreen Cancer Center, Evergreen Hospital, for being willing to share with generosity her extraordinary grasp of the many issues surrounding breast cancer; and for her time, energy, and resources.

To Elaine Lachlan, M.S.W., Social Oncologist, Wellness Works, Evergreen Cancer Center, Evergreen Hosptial, for her generous, insightful sharing of what happens to relationships in a breast cancer patient's life through this trauma; for the invaluable experience of allowing me to interface repeatedly with Bosom Buddies, a breast cancer support group through Evergreen Cancer Center—to listen, to learn, to become better informed regarding the daily challenges of women who face breast cancer.

To all the members of Bosom Buddies, a breast cancer support group at Evergreen Cancer Center, for allowing me to be present with them, to learn from each one as they shared from the heart what their individual journeys are; to witness the courage and support they offered each other—the rage and the joy of life they embrace.

To the breast cancer survivors who allowed me to interview, and/or accompany them on the very personal journey to radiation and/or chemotherapy treatment, and in some cases, be photographed during the process: Stephen Meredith, Debbie Collier, Kathryn Gunther, Trudy Bendix, Penny Schick, Evelyn Frazell, Sharon McKee, Teresa Martinez, Rebecca Maryatt, Susie Cornelius, and many others.

To Dr. Richard Clarfeld, Breast Cancer Surgeon, for allowing me to interview him regarding the incidence of minority women with breast cancer in his practice.

Dr. Bruce Neu, Plastic Surgeon, who offered invaluable perspective, credibility, and knowledge with respect to breast cancer reconstruction, the result of years of experience as a plastic surgeon.

To Dr. Richard Welk, Plastic Surgeon, The Polyclinic, Seattle, WA, who generously offered his time, enthusiastic energy, and knowledge regarding breast cancer reconstruction; to Pat Papadopulous, C.S.T., Dr. Welk's assistant, for her support of my efforts; and to the members of the Breast Reconstruction Support Group at The Polyclinic, for allowing me to visit and hear their experiences with breast reconstruction, observing firsthand the results of their surgeries.

To Dr. Erin D. Ellis, Tumor Institute, Swedish Medical Center, for sharing invaluable information regarding stem cell transplantation.

To Deborah Shiro, Program Manager, Detection, Washington Division, American Cancer Society, for contributing significantly to the "Network of Support" section.

To Dr. Gloria Mitchell, who opened my eyes to the added challenges facing minority women who deal with breast cancer.

To Liz Ilg and Patricia Van Kirk, who shared with me the particular challenges of lesbian women with breast cancer.

To Marion Lynch, M.D., A Fellow in Cancer Prevention, Fred Hutchinson Cancer Research Center, Seattle, WA, for reviewing "Lesbians and Breast Cancer."

To the following people who gave me a glimpse of how it is to support a breast cancer patient: Bill Baker, Patty McFee, Norma Plumb, Nikki Nordstrom, Dan Morgan, the staff at Wellness Works, Evergreen Hospice, and Evergreen Cancer Center, to name only a few.

To Sheryn Hara, marketing agent and coordinator of this project, thank you for believing in the value of this book and its message, and especially for being willing to undergird the success of this project with all you had available, your time, your energies, and your never-ending enthusiasm even when difficult challenges faced us in the process.

To Margaret D. Smith, editor, poet, and sculptor of the personal account, who offered her invaluable skills, insight, and enthusism.

To Susi Henderson, editor, who meticulously and artistically etched out the final form of the final book, even with numerous unforeseen challenges.

To Carol Lindahl, copy editor and proofreader, who, with extraordinary dedication, readied copy for publication.

To Ursula Bacon for creating a splendid cover; and to Thorn Bacon for creating a fitting title.

ACKNOWLEDGMENTS FOR BREAST CANCER CHARTS
"Stages of a Mastectomy" and "Shifting Relationships"*

To the original workshop participants and developers: first, the breast cancer survivors and Sandra Johnson, M.S.W., Supervisor at Evergreen Cancer Center, who helped create the original format for the "Stages of a Mastectomy" by digging deep into their personal memories and painful experiences in order to help others on their way. They created the original shape and content of these charts, and continued to contribute significantly, as they were able, as the charts emerged to their present form.

Kathryn Gunther, a warrior with a raucous sense of humor, a true individualist who stretched our thinking regarding who's in charge as a patient.

Florence Hannah, a proud grandmother, a person who embraced the painful experience of breast cancer and created something beautiful, which she shared with us all.

Tara Havemeyer, a brave warrior who died from breast cancer before this book was completed, but who inspired us all with her candor, strength, and great courage.

Sharon Harnden, a gracious human being who shared her challenges and reflections of courage from the heart.

Cora Hill, who was in the middle of chemo treatments and still came to share her pain and wisdom.

Annette Porter, who shared with us frankly how it was for her to make this journey, teaching us with photographs to honor the baldness she and others experience from chemo, transforming it into a thing of beauty.

Marie McClintock, who died of breast cancer one week before our first workshop—an honored warrior, her loving ways and courage heartened many of us on our way, and whose heart thoughts are present in this book.

Frenchie Williams, a brave, beautiful young woman, who shared her story with us from the heart.

Sandra Johnson, who shared with us her invaluable perspective as a cancer support person.

To the many people who contributed significantly to the development of the Breast Cancer Charts, the ideas of which are represented in this book, I extend my heartfelt appreciation for what it cost you to go back into the fire of the experience and pull out its meaning, thread by painful thread. By the reactions of the many people who have interfaced with the charts so far, I would say that your efforts have been much appreciated.

Judith H.M. Jones, B.S., Wellness Works, Evergreen Cancer Center.

Elaine Lachlan, M.S.W., Wellness Works, Evergreen Cancer Center, for contributing significantly to the groundwork for the "Shifting Relationships" charts.

Dr. June Strickland, Member of the Alaska Native/American Caucus, American Public Health Association, Consultant to the Office of Minority Health, NCI, Regional Outreach Coordinator, CIS (Cancer Information Service), NCI, Principal Investigator on a Southwest oncology national BSE study.

Georgiana Arnold, Health Care Professional, Project Director, the W. K. Kellogg Community-Based Public Health Initiative.

Elaine Dao, A.R.N.P., Director of Nursing Services, Kinon Nursing Home.

Carolina Lucero, Director, Home Care Division, SEA MAR Community Health Center, Seattle, WA.

Members of Bosom Buddies (breast cancer support group), Evergreen Cancer Center.

Liz Ilg, Head of Lesbian breast cancer project.

Patricia Van Kirk, breast cancer survivor.

Val Jean, breast cancer survivor.

Evelyn Frazell, breast cancer survivor.

Nikki Nordstrom, R.N.

Cancer survivors I have interfaced with in workshops, hospitals, health care centers, and individually over six years.

*These multi-cultural Breast Cancer Charts will be coming out in full form in 1995 as professional processing kits available to families and the medical community for assisting those who walk through the experience of breast cancer. "The Stages of a Mastectomy" and "Shifting Relationships" charts represent personal interfacing with about 75 breast cancer survivors, both formally and informally, as well as the input of a number of health care providers with many years of experience with breast cancer survivors. I would estimate, therefore, that the charts represent the experiences of approximately 2-3,000 breast cancer survivors: the women personally interviewed, plus the women whom the specialized health care professionals have observed through the years, and for whom they speak.

The reaction to the Breast Cancer Charts from breast cancer survivors, loved ones, health care professionals, and doctors has been extraordinary. A walk-through inter-active display with photographs, sculpture, and music is planned for 1995. For more information regarding these charts, or for a viewing of the display, write Clo Wilson-Hashiguchi, P.O. Box 12634, Bothell, WA, 98082. (*See* Order Form in back of the book.)

Contents

Stealing the Dragon's Fire
Clo Wilson-Hashiguchi

Part I
Dragon Nose

"Dragon Nose" is the name that spontaneously emerged for my breast cancer as I wrote shortly after I was diagnosed. The image that followed delighted me, mysteriously giving me back a sense of control. I found that, rather than an unformed mass of unknown terror, breast cancer become a named monster that I could rage at, mock because of the fun I had with its image, and fully acknowledge as a real-life dragon that stormed daily in my life, breathing fire and creating destruction. A stark metaphor, it offered me a vehicle with which to process the monstrous journey of breast cancer.

The dragon image seen in this book was created by my 16-year-old daughter, Monica, who has shared with us what that dragon looked like to her as a 10-year-old girl walking bravely beside a mother diagnosed with breast cancer.

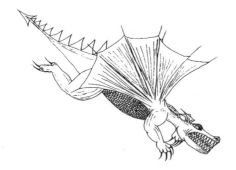

Introduction

What We Are Facing

I have written this book for each woman who finds herself facing this dragon of breast cancer.

You are incredibly unique, and so will your battle be with the dragon. Breast cancer is about people. It's not about numbers or medical facts or statistics. Breast cancer is about you and those who choose to walk through this nightmare beside you.

For the most part, breast cancer is about women, those who are facing the hard fact that they have somehow contracted a terrifying, potentially disfiguring, life-threatening disease.

In the United States alone, the American Cancer Society estimates 182,000 women will be diagnosed this year with breast cancer. Of those, 46,000 will die. Of eight women who live to be over 85, one will deal with this disease. These are not just statistics but mothers, daughters, sisters, grandmothers, friends—all loved ones.

It may come as a surprise that men, too, suffer from breast cancer, but at a much lower rate than women. The American Cancer Society suggests about 1,000 men will be diagnosed with the disease this year, and of those, 300 will die. Included in this book is an interview with a male breast cancer patient, who shared his insights about the experience.

Because men are not as aware that they need to check for this disease, it is usually found in a more advanced stage. Since for men there is not as much breast tissue, the spread of cancer from the breast tissue to other body tissues is typically more immediate and far reaching.

The questions regarding breast cancer are many, the answers few. For the patient, hearing a diagnosis of breast cancer is shocking. The treatment is often harsh. To compound this, the understanding of many of the medical staff regarding the psychological and emotional effects on the patient is abysmal. Then, for the female breast cancer patient, issues dealing with her identity as a woman must be addressed. These are different issues than if the cancer were found in another organ.

"I don't have a relationship with my liver or kidney," one vibrant 69-year-old breast cancer survivor relayed to a group of women, "but I do have a relationship with my breast." Losing a part of one's femaleness is a delicate issue that a woman with breast cancer must deal with repeatedly with the medical community and those close to her, if they are to understand her strong feelings about the matter.

In our society, a woman's breasts are often considered the most significant part of her valued femaleness. Even though breast cancer is so widespread, it may be hard for many men, even those who are cancer doctors (oncologists) to empathize with a woman's grief over losing such an integral part of herself.

Breast cancer is a real-life dragon, for which a battle plan for survival must be drawn up. One minute, life seems rather normal. The next, life is a deadly contest, where the breast cancer patient is buffeted from decision to decision, often with scanty information and certainly not enough medical background to feel very competent. Sadly, the medical community, supposedly a haven for the battle-weary patient, is often ignorant of the devastating emotional effect of breast cancer on the individual and her loved ones.

A well-respected plastic surgeon in the area of breast cancer once told me that there is a great variety of responses from women who go through a mastectomy. "Some patients," he pointed out, "have a much more difficult time than you did. For others, it is rather like getting a tooth extracted. They come in and go out of here with seemingly little effect on their lives."

Just for the record, in six years of listening to and interviewing women with breast cancer, I have yet to meet a woman who would equate having her tooth extracted with having her breast removed. His ignorance of the impact this has on the life of women was appalling to me.

As you will see from my story, I was fortunate enough to find a number of people in the medical community who were sensitive to my battle with the dragon. From my conversations with other breast cancer survivors, though, I discovered that many doctors only deal with "the tip of the iceberg"—the medical experience. Often these doctors are unaware of the torrent of reactions patients undergo, apart from the medical experience itself.

These reactions are borne out in the Breast Cancer Charts* created by breast cancer survivors and health care specialists. These people helped to record the stages of their journey through this disease, as well as the shifting patterns of relationships which they have lived through.

Typically, the patient will not share much more than medical information with her doctor. Only if she feels supported in this battle will the patient take what little energy she has left to share her mind and heart with her physician.

So, on the surface, it may seem to some doctors that the patient is handling everything calmly and rationally. Yet in this battle against a dragon, the patient's mind and emotions are raging. Outrageous visual images often come to mind to clarify, as dreams sometimes do, the meaning of this death-defying experience.

In the midst of a riveting diagnosis, a person must learn to be clear-headed. What is amazing is how clear we do become. How quickly we learn to forge the weapons we need to fight our battle. We take pains to arm ourselves well. We learn to trust our gut feelings. We develop our others who have battled this monster and won. We listen intently and fight hard.

Developing a raucous sense of humor offers us new perspective, which helps clear our minds and hearts. We take more time to honor what delights us: spending time with a child, climbing a mountain, dancing. We learn enormous patience. We learn to take naps. We learn to listen to our bodies in extraordinary ways. We learn how to heal. We learn to accept the unacceptable. And we learn to be thankful, very thankful, just to be alive.

A breast cancer survivor has battle wounds, sometimes quite disfiguring ones, sometimes not. At times the breast is gone entirely; sometimes there is only a small scar. Sometimes reconstruction is done to attempt to restore a sense of normalcy. But it is never quite the same.

There may be deeper wounds, more hidden, borne often with what appears to be a bit of sadness or even a touch of bitterness, and quite predictably, an ironic sense of humor. Fear is a companion well known and well respected among breast cancer survivors. We have learned a kind of irreverent dance with it. Among a group of breast cancer survivors there is often a sense of camaraderie, a sharing of battle stories and times of tears. Facing one's own mortality and personal disfigurement in the same battle tends to change one's perspective on how to live life, and perhaps even the choice of one's companions along the way.

There is new hope on the horizon. An incredible race for the cure of breast cancer has begun, largely due to the enormous pressure that breast cancer patients themselves have finally begun to apply together in significant places to heighten the public's awareness, and to loosen more funds for research. Thousands of breast cancer survivors have initiated support groups for those who accompany or follow them on this journey. Just knowing there are so many survivors gives those who come later the courage to try.

The medical and health care personnel who fight by our side, and the research scientists who aggressively search for the cause and cure of breast cancer need to be commended, and they deserve our strong support. When we figure out how to strike down this many headed monster once and for all, there will be celebration felt around the world comparable to any post-world-war celebration. There will be singing and dancing in the streets and on the mountain tops, in the churches and synagogues, in taverns and market places.

It will be wild and lovely. And there will be candles lit. Thousands of them, to honor those who have died on the battle front. Our goal is to arrive at a place where not another young girl or her family will ever worry about breast cancer. In the meantime, we are passing on to one another how to steal the dragon's fire.

*These charts are included in a kit being developed to help those who experience breast cancer personally or professionally. See the *Acknowledgments* for a more thorough description. You may request information using the *Order Form* in the back of the book.

"There are good doctors out there, ones who understand their role and *your* role—but you have to look."

— Annette Porter, breast cancer survivor

"Women need to take charge of their own health. The doctor is an advisor, not a God. When we don't even understand our own diagnosis, we don't have the means to go forward."

— Susie Cornelius, breast cancer survivor

"Don't wait around to see about any suspected problem. Have your doctor check it."

— Evelyn Frazell, breast cancer survivor

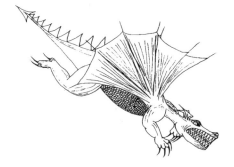

1

Mammogram

Panic—Too Early To Tell

Outside the Women's Clinic, the maples and ash were brilliant with their fall display of colors. Taking a deep breath of crisp air, I felt so alive!

But I hated these gynecological exams, and with five female-related surgeries in the past two years, I had had my share. But, if I had to have them, my OB, Dr. Asmussen, would be my first choice. He was always respectful and gentle.

On my walk down the hallway, I wondered what Doc would find, besides a very persistent yeast infection.

"That's the worst yeast infection I've seen in a while, but everything else looks good," he said after the examination. "Are you having any problems?"

"No, but we've had a pretty busy life, so I'm happy to hear everything is okay," I said with relief. "It'll be nice to have the yeast infection cleared up. It's pretty uncomfortable." A number of us in the family were recovering from a variety of ailments simultaneously. I was exhausted, both from my own surgeries and the illnesses of my family. But I felt sure things would soon be clearing up, with those major catastrophes seemingly out of the way.

There *was* another oddity going on, but I never thought to mention it. Any small cut or scratch during the past two months had been turning into a boil. No ordinary salve would touch it. In desperation, I had applied hydrogen peroxide, which seemed able to combat the problem. But Dr. Asmussen was an Ob/Gyn, not a family doctor, so I never thought to tell him.

"A breast check," he said as he looked over my chart. "Have you noticed anything new?" he asked.

"A bit of thickening in the left breast," I said as I scooted back on the examining table. I lay back on the small pillow.

"Hmmm. There is a thickening here. When did you notice this?" he asked.

"In the last month," I said casually. "It's quite painful. I've had fibrocystic* breasts for several years. Our family doctor, Dr. Dawson, suggested that I might be sensitive to the processing chemicals used in preparing coffee. I sometimes have breast pain within an hour of drinking a cup of coffee, so I seldom drink it."

"Have you ever had a mammogram?" Doc asked.

"No, I've been meaning to for a couple of years, but just haven't done it, with all of the surgeries."

"Well, I want you to have a mammogram to get this checked," he said with some concern. "And, even if it comes back all right, I'd like to schedule you for a biopsy within a month, just to make sure. Mammograms are only about 90 percent accurate." He leaned back on the counter, looking at me. "We fixed up the other problem. Now we need to take care of this."

"How do you do a biopsy?" I asked, thinking uncomfortably of the facial skin biopsies I had had on my lips and cheek.

"With a long needle," he said. "We numb the area, and then just put the needle in to take out some of the tissue to send to the lab."

"Well, I haven't done anything for excitement for a while," I joked, thinking of all the "cut and paste" that had just been completed on my body in the past couple of years. Just what I wanted—a biopsy!

I watched as he filled out the referral sheet for my next stop. *Breast lump, left breast.* It looked so final.

"Be sure and get the mammogram as soon as possible," he said. "You might even stop over today."

"Okay, Doc," I said cheerfully. "I'll take care of it." I gave him a hug. "Thanks."

"Don't forget," he said kindly.

"I won't," I said, thankful for this man who had been able to fix up my body—not without some complications—so that I could function normally again. Rectocele, cystocele, hysterectomy, and bladder repair—two hospital visits, and five surgeries.

As soon as I dressed, I found my way to the mammogram office next door. I gave the receptionist the referral sheet with the words, *Breast lump, left breast* on it. It evoked an odd sensation, as though the referral were for someone else.

"We happen to have an opening right now," she said cheerfully. "Would you like to stay and go in right now? Look," and she showed me her scheduling pad, "it's open!"

"Sure," I said. "Why not?"

"Do I need to take off my pearls?" I asked the technician as I stood, my upper half draped in a flimsy paper gown, slit down the front.

"Yes," she said.

"I guess it would add an interesting pattern to the pictures," I laughed. She walked me purposefully across the hall, into a room set up like a living room, except for a large metal apparatus on the right side. Intimidated by its size, I followed her carefully recited instructions.

"Put your right breast on this platform," she said. "I know it may be a little cold. There. Good. Just let me know if it hurts. I don't want to hurt you," she said with concern as she pressed my breast flat on the tray.

"Now, I need to press this down on your breast to get a good picture." She pressed a flat plastic plate down on the upper side of my breast, and secured it firmly. "It may be a little uncomfortable. I'm sorry. It will only be a moment."

My breast was well flattened between these two plastic presses in several different positions, one at a time. I thought of a pancake turner, pressing down on a hamburger frying in the skillet.

"It's wonderful to be a woman," I quipped to the technician as she stepped behind the machine to take the picture. "Men have no idea what they're missing."

"Yes, that's true," she said. Then a moment later her voice filtered back: "But they *do* have prostate exams."

"That's true," I said, but it didn't make me feel any better at the time. This lady I had never met before flip-flopped my breast between these two plastic plates, pressing and kneading my breast into the proper position. I detached myself from that breast on the platform, thinking of making cinnamon rolls, kneading the dough on a breadboard.

"A man must have designed this machine," I said. A woman, I figured, would have thought of something more comfortable, less intrusive. In the future, this will be done by something simpler, like sonar. For now, it's the best we have. But I don't have to like it!

After the mammogram, the technician asked me to sit on the couch and asked if I knew how to do a self-examination.

"Yes," I said confidently.

"Well," she said, "you may learn a few new things with this video. You can watch it while I go process the film." The video began to roll.

One in every 10 women today have breast cancer.

You owe it to your children and to your husband to get a regular check-up. You should do a self-examination every month, so that you can note any differences in the tissue. One in every 10 women... one in every 10... one in 10...

What if...The repetitive pounding of the video words seared my thoughts. What if that thickening was cancer? For the first time the possibility hit me. I tried to take a deep breath, but it caught short.

By the time the technician returned, I was no longer in the mood for laughing or joking. I was scared. I wanted to know, what if it really was breast cancer?

"Can you tell whether there is something to be concerned about?" I asked the technician seriously as she stood in front of me.

"I cannot discuss it. The doctor will go over the pictures with you," she said. All of a sudden, this pleasant, blond technician became like a robot to me, a mouth and a body with sounds coming out.

"When will I know?" I asked her.

"He will have them by Monday morning. We will send them over today. He will call you with the results."

Placing the pearls back around my neck, I walked out. As I headed toward the door, the technician handed me a white carnation.

White…pale…I had an urge to scream, but I didn't. I felt as if someone had just given me a carnation to put on my grave!

I wanted to drop the carnation, to get rid of it. But it seemed stuck to my fingers. I wanted to throw it far away from me, so we weren't connected in any way.

This was a thoughtful gesture, I tried to reason with myself. Why am I reacting this way? When I got out into the parking lot, I looked for a place to throw it. It embarrassed me that I felt this way about such a considerate gift. My daughter, Moni, would like it. She would enjoy its fragrance and bloom. Fighting the strong urge to destroy the flower, I placed it as far away as I could in the front seat and drove carefully home. I found a vase for it, put it quietly on Moni's study desk, then had to walk away.

By now, I was aware that something serious could be approaching our family. My palms were icy. What if? Oh God, no! With all of the other surgeries—not this, too! I tried to focus, to meditate. But an overwhelming panic surrounded me. Calm down, I told myself; you don't know for sure. It could be nothing, just a large cyst. There's no family history. I exercise regularly. I try to eat nutritious foods.

I tried to remember how refreshing and life-giving water feels, flowing over my body during my early morning lap swimming. The tension began to dissipate.

Father, Mother, Great Spirit: I know you are with me now, as you have always been. Please let me know your strength. Now I know why you have been urging me to get a mammogram—but there was so much going on with the other surgeries. I'm scared, but I know you care what happens. Help me with this.

*The term *fibrocystic* has become a catch-all phrase for a number of conditions that produce abnormal tissues in the breasts, mainly areas that feel firm, hard, or bumpy. Most of these are non-cancerous conditions. See *Part III: Breast Cancer Handbook* for more details.

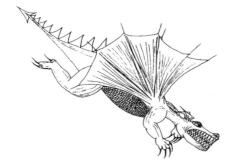

2

Breast Lump

Telling Friends and Family

When I heard Doc's message on my answering machine, I knew it was serious. I called back, hoping to hear that kind, familiar voice on the other end. Instead, his assistant came on the line.

"Your mammogram came back showing a lump of 2.5 centimeters," she said. "The doctor would like you to go to a surgeon for a biopsy. The doctor's name is Dr. Lennard, and his phone number is..."

Only 2.5 centimeters, I thought as I mechanically jotted down the number. It sounded quite small to me.

"He'd like you to call right away," the nurse was saying. I sensed the urgency in her voice. "Dr. Lennard is next door to us in the clinic. Just call and get an appointment."

"Okay," I said weakly. I felt like a hot potato, being passed from doctor to doctor.

After I hung up the receiver, my knees felt weak. It's possible that it's just a cyst, I tried to reassure myself. But still, I thought, a biopsy. I felt like a child, wanting to run away from the pain of the needles and the scalpel.

Where was that little booklet that my friend, Ellie, shared with me? It had a toll-free number to call, so I could be on their prayer list. I found it by my bed and dialed the number.* A man's voice answered.

"Silent Unity. How may I help you?"

"My name is Clo," I said, trying to control my feelings.

"Yes?" He waited.

"The doctor's office just called to inform me that I have a lump in my breast, and that I need to go in for a biopsy. They think there is a possibility it might be cancer..." The tears began to overflow as I spoke the dreaded word.

I could hear him in the background, reassuring me that God wanted me to be in perfect health, that healing would come, and that he and the rest of those in Silent Unity would begin praying for my complete recovery. His words ran together as the panic I felt rolled over me like an ocean wave. Sobbing, I could not respond as he spoke kindly, fully believing that this would find a positive solution. Just hearing his calm voice helped me. I felt peaceful.

The phone rang.

"Clo?" a familiar voice asked. "This is Dr. Asmussen."

"Yes," I said quietly, grateful to hear his steady voice.

"I thought you might be upset by the news. How are you doing?"

"It did come as quite a blow," I said, still wiping the tears from my cheeks. "I'll be all right."

"Dr. Lennard's a fine surgeon," Doc said. But, if you'd rather have another surgeon in the clinic, they are all very good."

"No, Doc," I said, his kindness touching me. "If you have recommended him, I'm sure he will be very good."

"Do you have any questions?" he asked.

"Two and a half centimeters. Is that large?"

"Yes," he said. "Dr. Lennard is a specialist in this area. He will know better than I what we are dealing with."

"Okay," I said. "Thanks for calling, Doc. I really appreciate it."

When the phone rang again, it was my friend, Pat. She and I were business partners, having built up a small business, a substitute teacher pool for private schools in the Greater Seattle Area. Pat wanted to know the results of the mammogram.

"I can't handle calling the surgeon today," I said. "I've just had so much cutting on my body, Pat."

"I understand how you feel, Clo. But you will call, won't you?" she said caringly. "You know you must call," she insisted.

"I know, Pat," I said. "But I need some time to get my bearings. I just can't handle it today."

"This is Monday. I'll call Wednesday to make sure you've called the doctor. Okay?" she asked. Her positive attitude made me smile. This is assertiveness in its best form, I thought.

"All right, Pat. Thanks. You're a dear."

"You'll be in my prayers, Clo," she said kindly.

When I got off the phone I went into the front bathroom, and looked at my breasts in the mirror—full and mature. Two babies had suckled them for food and comfort. They were such a part of my femaleness. They had been the source of much pleasure.

I remembered as a young girl growing up, standing in front of my bedroom mirror just like this, looking at my budding breasts, wondering if I'd ever have anything more than small buds. Now I wondered what was ahead.

"Glenn," I said at breakfast, "I could sure use one of those big, warm Gooch hugs this morning. I'm having a rough time with this."

"Gooch" had been the nickname his friends had given Glenn many years before I had known him. He called me "Willie."

He wrapped his strong arms around me, letting me soak up his warmth, then finished putting on his wool socks, one at a time, then his working boots, for another day's hard work in his gardening business.

I mechanically packed lunches for the kids. They were not yet aware there was something in the wind. I wanted to speak with the doctor first before deciding what to tell them.

"Mom! Mom, I need your help," Moni called from her bedroom. By the time I got there, she had already figured out the question she had about her homework.

I hustled our son Brian into the shower.

Cereal, bagels and freshly made warm applesauce. Get the kids out the door to catch the school bus…close the door.

I called my mother-in-law, Mitsuko, to let her know the results of the mammogram.

"Lots of women have it done," Mits said. "It's a good thing they caught it in time. You'll be fine, Cloey." I hardly heard her kind offer to help, not yet ready to hear such positive rhetoric. But I knew she would be there all the way. Being there for her family and friends was Mits' life.

Why was this so hard? I'd handled many difficult things in my life. Why did I feel like I was falling apart?

I dialed my mom's number. Ralph, her husband after my father died, answered.

"Well, hullo!" he answered in his deep rich voice. "Yes, I'm just fine. Gaining a little weight every day. I can't get over how long it takes to get well, though, Clo Ann. I suppose you can't expect anything else at 94. The old body just doesn't heal as fast, I guess."

He was proud of his longevity, and particularly proud of his good health.

"What do you think it is, Ralph?" I had asked him curiously at his 92nd birthday party. "What is it that has enabled you to live to a very healthy 92 years old, when others barely make it to 50?"

"Well," he said, cocking his weathered head as he spoke. "I take good care of myself. And, I drink two glasses of water—that's warm water, about the temperature of the body, so it isn't shocking—every morning when I get up—before I do anything else. You should do that, too, Clo Ann. My father taught me to do that when I was very young. He said it would keep me healthy. I don't think I've missed very many days. It helps clean out the body."

Since hearing his sage advice, I began drinking water in the morning, too. It certainly couldn't hurt, I reasoned, and it just might make a difference. It seemed so simple.

"How is your family?" he asked.

"Fine," I said. "Just fine. Can you have Mom call me when she comes in?"

"Sure," he answered. "I'll tell her you called."

"Thanks," I said bleakly.

I felt like I might burst from the raging emotion. I'll call Georgia, I thought. Just talking to someone who has gone through a mastectomy should help diffuse the emotion. It made me feel better just thinking of our warm-hearted, grandmotherly friend, who had "adopted" our kids, just as she had cared for many other children through the years. "I just love 'em," she'd say simply.

"Georgia? This is Clo," I said. "How are you doing?"

"Hi, Clo. I've been thinkin' about you," she said "How're the kids?"

"Fine," I answered. I hesitated. "Georgia, I just wanted to call to tell you I'm going in for a biopsy. They found a lump—2.5 centimeters, about one inch." There, it was out.

"Oh, no!" she said knowingly.

"I remember when you were going through this," I said. "I'm having a rough time with it. I just found out yesterday. I feel like it will all work out in the end, Georgia, but it's rough."

"I know just how you feel," she said softly. "I was the same way." With her comment, the tears began to run freely on my end of the phone. She understood. No false optimism. No "It'll be all right." Just sharing a feeling of fear of the unknown.

"My fear is not of cancer right now, Georgia," I said quietly, "but of having to go under the knife again. Pretty soon there'll be nothing left of me!" We both chuckled, then I added slowly, "I feel…violated, being poked and probed and cut so much. A real loss of privacy…"

"I know," she said quietly. "That's why I didn't go back for reconstruction. The gall bladder operation I had to have was so painful after having the mastectomy that I never went back to have the reconstruction done. Tom doesn't care. It's okay with him, so I'm not going to go through it."

"Thanks for talking with me, Georgia," I said, wiping my eyes dry. "It helps a lot just having someone else know what I'm feeling."

"I know," she said. "I'll be prayin' for you. Will you be all right?" she asked with concern in her voice.

"I'll be fine."

In fifteen minutes there was a knock on my door. When I opened it, there was Georgia, with her two young charges for the day.

"I thought you might need somebody with you this morning," she said simply. I let her loving arms come round me, as fear flowed out through my leaky eyes. Her granddaughter put her small arms around my legs, trying to help comfort me.

"What a sight we are," I laughed, as I recovered. "Come on in. I don't usually greet people by crying at the door."

I put on a pot of tea, and Georgia and I talked the morning away.

"We'll keep you in our prayers," Mom said when she called back. "It's going to turn out all right, Clo Ann," she said lovingly.

"Thanks, Mom," I said. "I feel it is, too. It's just working through it."

*A 24-hour prayer support service is available by calling
1-816-246-5400, or toll-free 1-800-669-7729
Or write: Silent Unity, Unity Village, MO 64065.

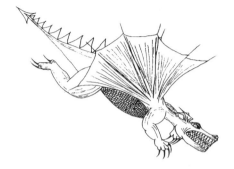

3

Consultation

Caring Partnership
with Doctor

I awoke calm, though very much aware of the impending consultation the following day. I began the outline of a new book and worked eagerly all morning.

In the afternoon I weeded for a long time in the rain. Growing up in Grays Harbor, Washington near the Olympic Rain Forest, I felt that the rain was my friend, not merely something to tolerate. Rain was familiar and refreshing. It grounded me.

It occurred to me as I yanked on the weeds that the lump might well have been the result of a build-up of stress over the past few years. I had observed through the many adventures of my life that my body seemed to play the role of shock absorber when mental or emotional stress ran too high. The signs of illness were a sure signal that I needed to assess what was going on in my daily life. I would then change course accordingly.

But this change of course was not always simple. There were a number of situations the past few years that spelled stress. First, Glenn had to get a new business off the ground, working around the clock.

Then there was the inevitable discomfort as I outgrew the skin of my old administrative job, deciding to write full-time and do workshops for area schools.

And there were the surgeries, as well as the ongoing celebrations and tragedies in our extended family.

Certainly there had been a number of things going on in our lives. I supposed there was cause for fatigue, after all.

Perhaps the stress had built up in my body, and my body was too much on overload to rid itself of it. I had felt a keen partnership with my body since I was a young girl and had to deal with hypoglycemia. But in the past few years I had lost touch. I was simply always tired, trying to find my way through the fog back to good health. There seemed to be just too many things to do, and never enough time or energy to do them. That kind of task-oriented thinking had to change. I promised myself that it would.

I took a moment to thank my body for the enormous effort it had put out in trying to regain its balance the past few years. I sent loving thoughts over and over to the lump in my breast, thanking it for taking on the extra stress of the past few years. Over and over I envisioned health being restored, first to that area, then to the whole of my body.

Feeling energized, I pushed a wheelbarrow full of weeds to the backyard and dumped it.

Waiting in the corner office for nearly an hour for the surgeon was chilling. Apprehensive to begin with, I sat in a hospital gown in the cold room, accompanied by a blowing fan. I had gone through all the magazines, and was starting again, when the doctor arrived.

"I thought you'd all gone home!" I said abruptly. He stopped momentarily and looked at me, taking in what I said.

"Sorry it's so cold in here," he said simply. "I am Dr. Lennard. And you are...Clo Hashiguchi."

"Yes."

"Dr. Asmussen referred you." As he perused my chart, he said, "You had a mammogram, and they found a lump of 2.5 centimeters."

"Yes," I said simply. I could sense his kindness through his comments, and was surprised how I felt immediately at ease with this man.

I sat up as he examined me. "This is very suspicious. It is an irregular shape," he said softly, as his sensitive fingers gently probed the tissues of my left breast. "And it is quite large. Usually we can begin feeling a lump at just one centimeter."

"How long do you think it has been growing?" I asked.

"Until we figure out what type it is, and even if it is malignant, we can't answer that. Maybe two years, maybe two months. With no history of cancer in your family, it is hard to figure." He stood back and looked at me.

"Its size makes me think we need to set you up for an appointment at the hospital."

The hospital! I thought. He thinks it will need to come out.

"But first, let's take a biopsy. Can you come in tomorrow?" he asked.

"Yes, I'll make arrangements," I said, surprised at the immediacy of the appointment.

"We will take a good sample, and take it right to the lab. Within 15 minutes we should have a pretty good idea of what we are dealing with," he said. "But, I will not make a final decision without the full lab report, which will come back by about next Tuesday."

I sat listening quietly as this gentle man began to talk about the possibility of malignancy, and possible chemotherapy and hormone treatment.

"I went through this with my family," he said. "One of the women had a mastectomy. So, I have some idea of how hard this is going to be for you to work through. I don't know personally, as a woman, of course. But I have some idea of what your husband will be going through. It will be hard on him. I will walk through this with you. We will work together for a cure."

Chemotherapy…a cure…what is he saying? He can't really be serious! My mind raced back to two good friends who had both died of cancer. My body turned to ice.

Then, I thought of my two good friends, Georgia and Pat. Five years ago Georgia had a mastectomy, and nearly twenty years ago, Pat. They were both doing great.

"For the biopsy, we will give you Valium and Demerol," he was saying. "And you should have someone pick you up. You won't be able to drive home. I will be taking a few days of vacation next week, so if we do need to make a hospital date, we'll make it after the Thanksgiving weekend."

Looking at this fellow human being who dealt daily in this arena, I said with feeling: "I'm sure you've earned a vacation."

We tentatively set the date for the hospital for the Monday following Thanksgiving. I went home with a deep sense that I was in a caring partnership with this doctor, and that he would do everything in his power to help me get well.

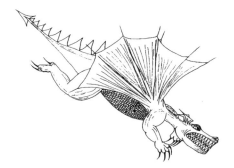

4

Biopsy

*Friends and Family
Offer Help*

The ring of the phone broke through the sounds of breakfast dishes clinking and the radio blaring out the local news. I wondered who was calling this time of the morning.

"Good morning, Clo. This is Karen. I'd like to take your kids today, and have them stay overnight. It's a perfect night for me." We often traded kids back and forth for sleepovers, much to their delight.

"Interesting you called," I said quietly. "I thought about calling you all day yesterday, wondering if you could watch Moni and Bri. I go in for a biopsy on my breast today, but I didn't want to bother you."

"Well," she said, "I just kept feeling I should call you and ask to have your kids come over today. Then Johnny came up to me this morning, and said, 'Mom, can Brian come over and stay all night?' I just laughed, and said inside, 'Okay! Okay! I'll call! I get the hint!' So I'm calling."

I thought of the other times Karen had been there for me at just the right moment.

Then she grew serious. "A biopsy," she said with concern. "How are you doing?"

"All right," I said, not really wanting to even think about it at that point. It was too close.

When the phone rang again, it was Ellie. "Clo," she said, "would you like me to come over this morning and be with you?"

"Thanks, Ellie. I'd love it!" I said. "The kids don't know anything yet, only that I'm going in to see the doctor this afternoon. It would make things a lot less stressful."

As Ellie and I shared a pot of tea, we talked about the ways we had both handled cancer before. Nothing I said or did shocked Ellie. She'd been there. Her daughter, Jan, had died recently of melanoma cancer, after years of fighting it valiantly.

"Jan was ready to go," Ellie said simply. In Ellie's written accounts of Jan's last days, Jan had voiced her struggle about whether she should keep fighting or let go and die. In the end, she let go and left the pain behind. Those who were with Jan before her departure felt that a spiritual healing had occurred, not only in Jan, but in themselves.

The skin cancer operations and the biopsies I had faced, plus the one I now was facing, paled by comparison to Jan's ordeal. Hearing part of her story again helped me with mine.

Ellie left several books that had helped her with Jan, including *Getting Well Again*, by Dr. Simonton, and *Anatomy of an Illness,* by Norman Cousins.

"I'm reading Bernie Siegel's book, *Love, Medicine and Miracles*," I grinned. "It's my homework for this weekend."

"That's good," Ellie smiled. "That will help. I feel everything is going to be all right."

"I do too, Ellie," I said. "I *must* find a way through this."

"How are you doing, Cloey?" Mits asked affectionately as she wove through the traffic. Mits was always there if anyone in the family needed her. She was a great support at this moment, driving me to the doctor's for the biopsy. Cancer's devastating enough when support is available. What do people do who don't have that support? I thought. I felt great empathy extended to those unknown people without friends and family to see them through.

"I'll just be glad when I know for sure, one way or another," I said softly. "Having had other biopsies, I know what I'm up against, and I'm not looking forward to it. It's not a bit comfortable." By four o'clock I should know, I thought. It'll be over, this waiting.

The nurse snapped a plastic identification band around my wrist, and once again I put a white paper hospital gown on top, slit open in the front. My body felt chilled.

Linda, the surgical nurse, went over the procedure with me, in a kind, unhurried way. I joked about anything I could, trying to defuse my nervousness. When we finished, she walked me into the surgical room, and over to the metal surgical table. We talked about our families as she prepped me for the doctor and inserted the IV.

When Dr. Lennard arrived, he and Linda exchanged information and set to work. I was surprised to feel my body shaking.

"I feel fine. I don't know why I'm shaking." I exclaimed to Linda, as the doctor prepped for surgery.

"It's okay, Clo. It's normal to be a little nervous." She made sure a warm blanket was tucked around my legs. Just having her there helped me as Doc painted the area he would be cutting into with a pungent yellow substance.

To Dr. Lennard I said, "Our family doctor, Dr. Dawson, said to relay to you that he would like to assist in surgery, to 'put in his two cents worth.'"

I had called Dr. Dawson's office to let him know about the biopsy that morning, feeling that he was part of our "family" who should be informed. Within fifteen minutes Doc had called back to share his concern, offering to be there at the surgery.

"That'll be great," Dr. Lennard responded, as he numbed the area. "Yes, I know Dr. Dawson," he said. Then his eyes twinkled. "Do you know what I like about you? Your eyes! Look at the color of mine." He turned slightly so I could get a better view.

"Green!"

"Those of us with these eyes must stick together." he said, laughing easily. I chuckled in spite of myself, warmed by his quick sense of humor.

"How are you doing?" he asked.

"I feel very thankful," I said reflectively. "I have a wonderful family and very supportive friends who are helping me through this."

"You're lucky," he said. "Not everybody does."

"How do they ever handle it?" I asked, thinking of the emotional roller coaster I had been on all week.

"It's very hard," he answered.

As he cut deeper and deeper into my breast, Linda continued to pass him surgical instruments and swabs. The area was bleeding profusely by the time he had sliced into the tumor. Both of them worked together as he cauterized the vessels to try to stop the bleeding.

"How does it look?" I asked, wondering what he was seeing with his experienced eyes.

"It looks very suspicious," he answered, continuing to work. "Tumor tissue is difficult to stop bleeding, and you can see, this is bleeding quite a bit." I could smell the singed flesh as he worked. Once in a while I could feel a small bite of pain as they worked, and he would stop to increase the numbness.

"I think I'd rather be in surgery, than have a biopsy," I said, as he took out the specimen for the lab.

"It's easier for me, too," he said. "It's such a small area to work in. With a mastectomy, it's a larger area. It's easier to control the bleeding."

They began stitching up the wound. "We want to keep it from bleeding any more," he explained, "so it doesn't go into the other breast tissue. Otherwise it will be harder during surgery, trying to get a clean specimen for lab analysis."

Four stitches were made across the incision to hold it closed, and a large bandage was applied.

I looked at the doctor. His eyes were bloodshot, and he looked tired. I wondered how cancer doctors deal with this every day.

"Now, Clo," he said, stepping back from the table, "the complete lab report will be in by Tuesday. We'll know in fifteen minutes what we're dealing with, but I wouldn't want to go any further without the complete lab report."

"What does it look like, Doc?" I asked.

"It looks very suspicious," he repeated. "It has the hard surface, and the inside is vascular. I'm pretty sure of what we're dealing with, but I'm going over to the hospital and will have them call you back. Linda will explain what happens next. We'll have you come back Monday to have this wound checked, then we'll schedule you for surgery next Monday morning."

He explained the mastectomy surgery in detail, the breast removal first, then the lymph nodes. "The cuts will be here and here," he explained, pointing to the areas on my chest. "I take this flap up and this one down. The first objective is to get out all these cancerous cells. The second is to save enough tissue for reconstruction, with as little damage as possible."

As he was cleaning up after the surgery, he added, "You're a great lady. You have a great attitude, a good support system, and you are mentally and emotionally stable. You're going to make it just fine."

I chuckled, thinking of what fun Glenn would have with the "mentally and emotionally stable" part.

"What about reconstruction?" I asked.

"You are a great candidate for that, Clo. I'm already going to plan on that for you." He readied himself to leave as we continued our conversation.

"What about the nipple, Doc?" I'd never thought about it before, but talking reconstruction made me wonder.

"It's pretty amazing what they can do," he answered. "They take a bit of the tissue from your other nipple, and build a new nipple with it."

"Oh!" I said. "That's incredible."

"Now, if you have any questions at all, I want you to call me. I know this won't be easy, so don't hesitate to call if it starts getting out of hand."

Linda helped me into my bra, which acted as a support for the bandaged breast, and walked me back to the examining room. She helped me lie down on the examining table to rest for a while, then left the room. I felt elated that I had completed the first phase of this adventure.

When Linda returned, she came over to me. "It came back positive, Clo," Linda said gently.

"Ohh," I said. A cold knot tightened in the pit of my stomach. "Malignant," I said more to myself than to her. She walked over and put her arm around my shoulder.

"So," I said weakly, "I go into the hospital the Monday after Thanksgiving. Happy Thanksgiving."

She waited quietly for the news to sink in. I could feel the tears beginning to come, so I took a deep breath.

"Okay," I said with difficulty. "Where do we go from here?"

Linda carefully took me through the schedule of events for the next week: check back for the biopsy on Monday, blood tests for the hospital surgery, possible check-in times.

I was in shock. This is really happening, I told myself. I have a malignant tumor. I'm going into the hospital again, this time to take out cancer. If they don't take it out, I will die.

"Would you like me to tell your mother-in-law?" Linda asked gently. "She's waiting in the lobby." She waited patiently as I thought about it.

"No," I said, thinking of Mits, and how tender-hearted she was. I needed to tell her to soften the blow. "I will tell her. But, thanks, Linda."

Then I asked her, "Will you be there with Dr. Lennard in surgery on Monday?"

"It's not my normal scheduled day," she said, "but I'll see if I can change my schedule around. Maybe I can."

I gave her a hug. "Thanks, Linda."

"Good luck, Clo," she said kindly.

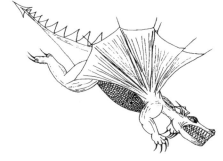

5

Diagnosis: Malignant
Tired but Peaceful

"Did you read all the magazines, Mits?" I said, kidding her. She looked worn out, waiting so long.

"I sure did." she quipped. "I read them all once, and now I'm reading them all again." Then she asked anxiously, "What did the doctor say?"

"It's malignant, Mits," I said quietly.

"Oh, no, Cloey!" she said softly. "Well, it's good that they found it out now. At least they can do something about it. They can take it out, right?"

"Yes," I answered carefully. "They will take the breast, and the lymph nodes under the arm, just to make sure."

"Make sure of what? They think that's all there is, don't they?" I looked at her worried eyes.

"I'm sure that's all there is," I said reassuringly. The thought that the cancer might have spread had not yet hit me, and I preferred not to explore the possibilities.

The numbness had not yet worn off, but still, the wound was uncomfortable. There was pain medication to take later on. For the time being, I was just glad to be going home.

"You go lie down and rest," Mits said as we walked in the house. "I'll make dinner." We had been through this so many times before. With my frequent jaunts to the hospital the past couple of years, Mits was always there to help, and by now she had our house routine down to a science.

I wondered if I'd ever be healthy enough to take charge of my own home again. Having to lie down while others cleaned my house, baked the chocolate chip cookies, and comforted my family was unbearable at times. I missed staying up with Glenn, enjoying an evening together. It had been a long time.

I had made it through the biopsy. That was step one. But as I sat on the bed, I suddenly felt more tired than I had ever been, and I cried.

Father, I am so tired. I can't fight anymore. I can't take any more pain. I appreciate all you've shown me in life. We've had many adventures together. You were always there with me. But I can't handle a mastectomy, the pain of another surgery, and cancer. I need the strength to fight it. There's nothing left. Just let me slip away.

The tears cleansed me as they helped me speak openly. It would be such a relief—no more battles, no more pain, no more sickly wife and mom, no more of this dark, heavy fatigue.

As I cried, I felt a gentle inner nudging, and a mental picture of each of my children began to emerge, like a delicate sprout reaching for the spring sun. The love I had for each of them began to warm me, like a fire on a wintry night. And then, a picture of Gooch, and the tenderness which had grown for him through the years.

Okay, I understand. I can see that I love them very much. But you're going to have to be there to help, because I have nothing left.

A deep peace settled over me. I felt surrounded by love. Tired, but with a new sense of purpose, I lay back down on the bed and fell asleep.

When I awoke, Mits had left, and Glenn had just arrived home from his landscaping work. We stood in the kitchen.

"What did they find?" he asked me tiredly.

"Glenn, it doesn't look good," I said, starting to choke up.

"Oh, no!" he said, dropping his head. I leaned against the stove, and he sat down heavily in a kitchen chair. He began to untie the laces on his work boots.

"Gooch," I said quietly, "I feel that this is going to work out all right in the end. Right now I feel like Bilbo Baggins in *The Hobbit,* trying to find a way through the mountain." I hesitated for a moment. "We've been through rough things before, but we have each other, and when things like this happen, the really important things seem to come forth very clearly."

He was sitting still, just listening.

"We are on an upswing," I tried to reassure him. "Our marriage has improved, and our finances are getting better and better. I feel like this cancer is a big piece of 'garbage' that developed from the past ten years of stress. Once it's gone, it will be a relief."

I shifted my weight and sighed as I leaned against the stove. "Dr. Lennard, the surgeon, has gone through this before with someone in his family."

"Is that right?" he asked, surprised.

"Yes. He said he has some idea of what we will be going through. He said he knew what you as the husband will be going through, too. Oh, you know what else he said?" I grinned. "He said that I am a great lady, I have a great attitude, and I am mentally and emotionally stable."

"Is that right?" he said in mock disbelief, smiling.

"What words could possibly describe the emotions you feel when someone tells you you have cancer? Stark fear and extreme sorrow. As each day passes, it becomes easier to think about dealing with the hand that is dealt you. I think the most important thing is that life without love is empty."

— Penny Schick, breast cancer warrior

"Breast cancer has made me realize I'm vulnerable. I used to believe I was not vulnerable to sickness and disease."

— Sharon McKee, breast cancer survivor

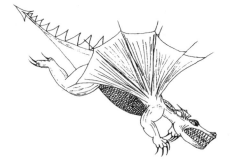

6

Preparation for Surgery

Life Goes On

The weekend dragged on like a very long stage play. Time seemed to stretch out in slow motion, with significant figures walking through their parts in a predetermined plot.

From the bedroom I could hear the chatter between Monica and Mits in the kitchen, dishes clinking in the sink, someone clunking down the steps to get the laundry, and the door slamming as someone came in from picking up the mail. I knew that Monica would be a great help for Mits and Glenn. Since she was a little girl, her strengths have come forth in crisis.

"Here, Mom," Moni said cheerfully, as she brought me in a cup of hot steaming tea.

"What a nice surprise!" I exclaimed, as she fixed a place to set it on my lap. "Thank you, Moni." I reached out my right arm to her to give her a somewhat awkward hug. "Mmmm. This tastes so good!" She beamed as she bounced out of the room.

"Does it hurt, Mom?" asked Brian, walking in quietly. He stretched out on my bed, looking at the wrap around my chest, his long legs dangling over the edge.

It isn't very comfortable," I said frankly, "but the pain pills help a lot."

"Will it hurt if I give you a hug?" he asked solemnly, his soft brown eyes searching mine.

"I would love one of your hugs," I responded. He rolled off the bed, landing solidly on both feet, and ambled over to the side of my bed. He wrapped his small young arms gently around my shoulders, trying not to hurt me, as he leaned his head against mine, his warm cheek touching my tired face.

"Thank you, Bri," I said with feeling. "That helps more than you know."

"Why did the doctor have to cut you?" he asked simply, surmising what happened from seeing the bandages on my chest.

"Well," I answered, trying to sound confident, "Doc is checking out a spot that showed up last week in a mammogram, an X-ray of the breast." He listened carefully as I tried to explain. "There's a small growth in this breast," I said, pointing to my bandaged left side. "They're trying to decide what they need to do with it."

"Will you have to go to the hospital?" he asked, worry creeping into his voice. He'd been this route before, and didn't like it.

"It looks like it, Bri," I said.

"I don't want you to ever die, Mom." Children seem to sense the truth, even when we try to protect them.

"One day I will," I said truthfully, "but not with this, Bri. I have lots to live for: you and Moni…and Dad." I said this with as much confidence as I could muster.

I watched Brian move through the doorway and began to pray.

Father, thank you for this family, and especially for the love we have for each other. Thank you for your love for me as I walk through this darkness. Hold my hand firmly. I don't want to get lost. Thank you.

"You need to reach out to those who are willing to help you, Clo," Ellie advised me one morning over coffee.

"That's hard for me, Ellie," I said. "It's different when I'm offering help to someone else, but to have to ask for help."

"I know it's hard," she persisted, "but you will need the help, and they will be glad you asked. It's part of your getting well."

I was feeling exposed, vulnerable, like a small child in an empty room. Asking for help would bring others into that cold, lonely room with me. My instinct was to crouch down, wrapping my arms tightly around myself, keeping all hurtful things out. To shift my frame of reference to extend myself, exposing my vulnerability, was terrifying.

On the other hand, I trusted Ellie's judgment. She had been through this before.

So I began to set the stage. "I will be going in for a mastectomy on the 28th," I relayed to family and friends, one at a time, as I was able to handle the calls. "Please send me only positive thoughts. Don't send us any negative thoughts—we don't need them. Think of what we might do together when we are through with this adventure. How we can celebrate. Please remember my family. This is very difficult for them, too."

As an administrator of a Montessori school for several years, I had implemented the technique of creative visualization. In personal and professional goal-setting each year, we identified an image of where we would like to be, then took the first practical steps in that direction. Even in working out sticky problems, if we could find an image of resolution, we would almost immediately see some results.

I had seen what creative visualization had done for each staff member's growth. I was a believer in its impact, and immediately set out to use what I had learned in this new arena—my survival of cancer.

As I made a cup of tea one afternoon, I got the feeling that I needed to review my relationships with friends and family for any rough spots. Somehow these would have the potential of clogging up the channel to healing. Making a mental inventory of my relationships, I came up with one that contained some unresolved hurt feelings. Quickly I took out a notecard, wrote a personal message to my friend, and had it delivered that day. It was a relieving, though curious, exercise.

"The initial news caught me by surprise. But afterwards, everything moved rather quickly. Right now, I'd say I was in a state of mental healing."

— Frenchie Williams, breast cancer survivor

"Put a woman in a situation where she can't duke it out, where she knows something's wrong, and she's helpless. Her hands are tied. She thinks through her options, and there's nothing she really can do. It's then that the body creates those bad cells."

— Cora Hill, breast cancer survivor

"Attitude is where it's at. A positive attitude goes a long way."

— Trudy Bendix, breast cancer survivor

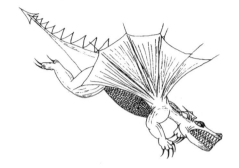

7

Reading about Healing

Stress—a Risk Factor

A number of years ago, when I had surgery for skin cancer, the surgeon told me that my type of skin cancer would never transfer to other parts of my body. But I was aware that my body *could* develop cancer when it was vulnerable, so I gave some serious thought towards understanding why it had occurred. I also worked on becoming informed on how I could prevent it happening to me again.

"You know, Doc," I said as the cancer surgeon finished stitching up the wound on my face, "I think this happened because of a great deal of stress that has occurred in my life over the past couple of years. I've always been very healthy, but there've been a few heavy-duty things that have happened recently."

He stood back from the table and rolled his eyes, peering at me and sighing.

"No, I'm sure it isn't stress," he said patronizingly. "We don't know why some people get cancer while others don't, but it is definitely *not* stress." He was obviously uncomfortable with me as a patient offering any suggestions as to why this had happened. He finished scrubbing his hands, and left the room.

I thought of the miscarriage the year before I had had Monica. The loss had been devastating. Glenn, a chemist, was working long hours as a quality control manager and was on call twenty-four hours a day. We were both stressed out and over-extended. I wondered why this doctor was uncomfortable listening to my assessment of why the miscarriage had happened. I was very much in tune with what went on in my body and I was sure stress was a factor, but I said no more.

Personally and professionally, I am research-oriented, and would never have given up the possibility of a new piece of evidence. I had seen similar close-mindedness in my own profession, education, and knew better than to waste any more of my analysis on this doctor.

The day after the biopsy for the breast lump, I reached for the copy of *Love, Medicine and Miracles,* by Bernie Siegel, sent by my friend, Carolyn. I flipped through the pages, hoping to light on something helpful.

"For the first time, I began to understand fully what it's like to live with cancer, knowing the fear that it may be spreading even while you talk to your doctor, do the dishes, play with the kids, work, sleep, or make love. How hard it is to keep one's integrity as a human being with this knowledge!"

That's how it is, I sighed. He's put my feelings onto the page.

"Exceptional patients refuse to be victims. They educate themselves and become specialists in their own care. They question the doctors because they want to understand their treatment and participate in it. They demand dignity, personhood, and control, no matter what the course of the disease…It takes courage to be exceptional."

The case of Mr. Wright, who had advanced lymphosarcoma caught my eye. He was so riddled with cancer tumors and complications in his internal organs that the doctor had given up, giving him medication as a sedative to ease the pain in his dying.

Mr. Wright had heard about a new drug called Krebiozen, which was to be evaluated at the hospital where he lay. He begged the doctor to give it to him. The doctor finally gave him one injection on Friday, thinking he would probably be dead, anyway, when he returned on Monday. But he was anything but dead!

"I had left him febrile, gasping for air, completely bed-ridden. Now, here he was walking around the ward, chatting happily with the nurses, and spreading his message of good cheer to any who would listen. The tumor masses had melted like snowballs on a hot stove. He had had no other treatment outside of the single 'useless shot.'"

In ten days, with continued treatment, Mr. Wright was discharged from his "deathbed," soon flying his own plane with no discomfort. However,

"...within two months, conflicting reports began to appear in the news, all of the testing clinics reporting no results...This disturbed Mr. Wright considerably...He was...logical and scientific in his thinking, and he began to lose faith in his last hope... After two months of practically perfect health, he relapsed to his original state and became very gloomy and miserable."

The doctor decided to take unusual action, to tell his patient that the early shipments "had deteriorated rapidly in the bottles," but that he had a new "super refined, double-strength product" which he could make available to Mr. Wright. Mr. Wright agreed to try the treatment, and the doctor injected, with great fanfare, what the patient thought was Krebiozen, but was really only fresh water.

His second recovery was even more dramatic than the first. For two months he remained symptom-free, with continued injections of only fresh water. But within days of a published report by AMA that Krebiozen was "a worthless drug in the treatment of cancer," he was readmitted to the hospital and succumbed within two days.

The case of Mr. Wright gave me concrete evidence that what I was about to attempt personally was possible. I could have physical control over the outcome of this disease, if I could only figure out in time what my own body needed.

Some years back I worked as a computer programmer. We were trained to be thorough and precise in our analysis. Otherwise, the program turned out to be useless. "Garbage in—garbage out," was the slogan we used, meaning that if wrong information is fed to a computer, wrong information will come out.

I felt like I was back at the computer, trying to decode a new computer language in time to meet a scheduled deadline for a customer. This time that customer was me, and "garbage in" could be fatal.

I went back to Siegel's book to search for clues that might help me as I prepared for the journey ahead. He goes on to say:

"The state of the mind changes the state of the body by work-ing through the central nervous system, the endocrine system, and the immune system. Peace of mind sends the body a 'live' message, while depression, fear, and unresolved conflict give it a 'die' message."

I collected this evidence, stacking it up piece by encouraging piece, building a sturdy frame of reference, in which I could operate as I prepared myself for the rough times ahead.

"Healing is not a coincidence… On the contrary, healing is a creative act, calling for all the hard work and dedication needed for other forms of creativity."

"Participation in the decision-making process, more than any other factor, determines the quality of the doctor-patient relationship. The exceptional patient wants to share responsi-bility for life and treatment, and doctors who encourage that attitude can help all patients heal faster."

I determined to share in the responsibility of every future deci-sion regarding my recovery, just as I had up to that point. I would not relinquish that privilege, nor the responsibility that accompanied it. I realized just how fortunate I was to have doctors who were willing to share that responsibility with me. I read on:

"Stress can be measured. One of the yardsticks for it...uses a list of 43 stressful changes to assess a person's likelihood of becoming ill. The evaluation begins with a history of the person's recent emotional life, then assigns a certain number of 'points' to each life crisis."

*"The highest [point] value... is attached to the most griev-ous loss, the death of one's spouse. This most traumatic of events is often followed by cancer or other catastrophic illness in one or two years...**Within one day** any uncontrollable stress lowers the efficiency of the body's disease-fighting killer cells."*

Like a window opening to let in new light, I "opened myself up" to understand what had caused the tumor. Then I tried to find just how I could help to get rid of the cancer and its side effects. Once it was gone, I reasoned, I could then work on prevention, so that no other cancer would occur.

I picked up Simonton's book, *Getting Well Again*. I wondered what additional ammunition he could offer me.

"There is a clear link between stress and illness, a link so strong that it is possible to predict illness based on the amount of stress in people's lives. Recent studies... suggest that the effects of emotional stress can suppress the immune system, thus shackling the body's natural defenses against cancer and other disease."

Simonton's work substantiated that a patient's frame of mind has a great impact on the success or failure of his recovery.

After a while I picked up the copy of Norman Cousins' *Anatomy of an Illness*, which Ellie had loaned to me.

Norman Cousins was the unfortunate victim of a serious collagen (connective tissue) disease. The chances of recovery given to him were one in five hundred. With those odds against him, and his doctors unable to give him any hope, he realized that if he were to get well, it would be up to him to take the initiative.

Having read substantially in the medical field, he began to ask some unorthodox questions of his doctor. If negative emotions have a negative chemical effect on the body, is it possible that positive emotions would have an equally positive chemical effect?

Is it possible that another environment, such as a hotel room, without all of the interruptions of a hospital room, would be more beneficial to a recovery? And, if vitamin C is known to have a positive effect on the immune system, would a slow, continuous intravenous drip help the body to utilize higher dosages through time, increasing his chances for recovery?

What did they have to lose, with such a bleak prognosis? So, with the full support of his physician, he began his radical program, choosing a hotel room in which to carry it out. High dosages of ascorbic acid were administered through a slow intravenous drip.

The final part of his plan was to set up a "program calling for the full exercise of the affirmative emotions as a factor in enhancing body chemistry." In other words, laughter indeed could be the best medicine. *Candid Camera* producer, Allen Funt, sent him some of his classics, and some old Marx Brothers films were ordered. They pulled the blinds on the windows and began to watch.

"It worked. I made the joyous discovery that ten minutes of genuine belly laughter had an anesthetic effect and would give me at least two hours of pain-free-sleep... Sometimes, the nurse read to me out of humor books. Especially useful were E.B. and Katherine White's Subtreasury of American Humor *and Max Eastman's* The Enjoyment of Laughter."

The positive emotions of "love, hope, faith, laughter, confidence, and the will to live" were fully implemented in the hotel room. Cousins recovered. He cited a trip he made to Dr. Albert Schweitzer's hospital in Lambarene, Africa. In discussing the role of a doctor of medicine compared with a local witch doctor, Schweitzer pointed out:

"The witch doctor succeeds for the same reason all the rest of us succeed. Each patient carries his own doctor inside him. They come to us not knowing that truth. We are at our best when we give the doctor who resides within each patient a chance to go to work."

I glanced at a small placard I had hung on the wall:

Limits exist only in the mind.

You're going to have a chance to discover if that is really true, or not, I reflected. Where is the *source* of this healing power? Where is it located…exactly? If I could know that, and be receptive enough, perhaps, I'll make it home free in time. On the other hand, perhaps it is in *letting go* that this human body is most empowered to regenerate itself. Will I know enough in time to make the difference?

Then I knew. I will simply act *as if* everything will turn out all right, and do everything I can to make that a reality. The rest is up to the Universe. Perhaps that's what an "act of faith" is really all about.

"You don't always have to be brave! It's okay to be angry! Let those around you fill you with love, hope, and a belief that you *can* beat this."

> — Priscilla McCarty, breast cancer survivor

"Breast cancer is not the worst thing in the world. We need to push back the horror of it and regain our humanness."

> — Patricia Van Kirk, breast cancer survivor

"Don't give up!"

> — Thomas S. Dawson, D.O., family physician

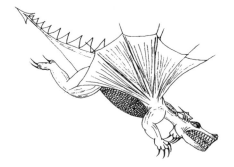

8

Friends Tell Their Cancer Stories

Spiritual Support

One of the side benefits in life is to be able to introduce interesting people to each other. On the day after Thanksgiving, Ellie invited Pat and me to her beautiful home so that we could talk over what was happening before I entered the hospital. These two extraordinary women were able to meet for the first time. Together we discussed very serious issues, sharing personal experiences and joining hearts.

Ellie told Pat about her daughter, Jan, who had died of cancer not long before, and she explained how the experience had enriched their family, despite the tragedy of losing her.

Pat told us about her own mastectomy as a young mother. Her doctor discovered a very small lump when she went to check out what she thought was an infection in her breast as a young nursing mother. With his discovery, the doctor advised her to come back in four hours to check into the hospital for a mastectomy.

"Four hours later!" I gasped.

"In some ways," she mused, "it was probably easier than what you are going through. I didn't have much time to think about it. I had to make arrangements for my sons. We went to church where I emotionally prepared for any eventuality." She sat quietly, remembering. "It was a shock, though. I remember thinking that if I had cancer, I just wanted to get rid of it."

I looked at my business partner with new eyes.

"I never knew," I said quietly.

"I know," she responded. "I thought it might help you, to know I had been through it. It's been almost twenty years. I'm doing great! I had a reconstruction done about two years ago, and I'm fine. My right side is looking more normal now."

"We'll be a matched pair," I chuckled. "Mine is the left side."

"Clo!" she laughed, her brown eyes dancing.

It was a pleasure, being part of an exchange among very positive women who were dealing with cancer.

After a while the conversation shifted to a different plane. Pat began talking about time as we know it being seen as a limitation to us. Suddenly I was overcome with a very strong sense of a shift of time, as though someone had opened a window to the future. I was sitting there, looking back on what was happening in the room. The feeling was disorienting and very strong. I decided to share my sensations with my friends.

"This sounds crazy," I said, "but I feel like the operation *has already been completed*, and that we are like actors in a play, just walking through our parts. This is crazy!" I repeated. "It's like what we are doing here has already occurred."

"Interesting," Ellie smiled. She had seen a lot of unusual happenings dealing with her daughter's illness. Nothing shocked her.

As the conversation continued, I sat on the couch as if in a time warp, unable to shake the strong sensation that *all was well on the other side of this operation*. It was oddly comforting.

Father, I know these two friends have been placed in my life partially to assist me with this cancer. They have been such a joy to me. Thank you. I remember telling them that I felt I was on a chess board, and people were being moved into place around me. As long as a year ago, I wondered what you were up to. You seemed to be making careful, deliberate preparations. Actually, it was fun to try to figure out what was up. Now, I know. Thank you for caring so much. Amen.

"I worry about living to see my 13-year-old son grow up. I worry about my son worrying about me. I have worked to fight this disease. Breast cancer has made me angry. I have become active in the public fight against it."

— Rebecca Maryatt, breast cancer survivor

"[O]ne's breasts are very personal and emotional parts. The loss is both a physical and an emotional one. Even knowing, after the diagnosis of cancer, that its existence is life-threatening does not diminish that emotional loss. And it certainly must be much harder for a younger woman."

— Florence Hannah, breast cancer survivor

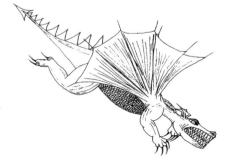

9

Into the Hospital

Fear

Up very early, I was surprised how refreshed I felt. With brush in hand I fluffed my hair from the perm Jill, my sister-in-law, had given me a few days before, misting it with a bit of hair spray. A coiffure to go into surgery? What peculiar creatures we are, I mused. I finished packing the last items, including toothbrush and toothpaste, and took a minute to update my journal. I could hear the familiar sounds of Mits stoking the fire in the wood stove.

"Good morning! Time to get up!" I sang out softly to my children. They stirred and grunted under their warm covers, resisting the early morning call. I padded into the kitchen, where Mits was bustling with the business of getting my family ready to meet the day.

"How you doing this morning, Cloey?" Mits asked, concern lacing her words.

"Fine," I said, "but last night was tough getting to sleep."

She poked the last sandwich into a bag, and I passed her a cereal box from a high shelf to complete the breakfast table.

Suitcases stood ready at the top of the staircase. I walked down the hallway to awaken Glenn.

"The kids are awake," I said, "and breakfast is on the table. It's all yours, now."

"Okay. Good luck, Willie," he said sleepily. "See you tonight."

"Thanks," I said, choking up. "I love you, Gooch," bending down to give him a hug.

"I love you, too, Willie."

The night before, dark rain clouds had filled the skies, the rain rhythmically pelting the rooftop as I lay in my bed trying to go to sleep. But this morning, a breathtaking pink and white sunrise rose to meet us as we drove down the hill, taking our familiar path to the hospital.

"We should always come this early," I quipped as we drove into the hospital parking lot. "There's a parking place right up front!" Mits looked at me sideways, laughing nervously.

"Good morning!" a cheerful grey-haired receptionist greeted us. She asked me the final questions, completing the necessary paperwork, then locked an ID bracelet firmly around my wrist. This is real, I said to myself. I am going in today for cancer surgery. I took a deep breath, trying to orient myself.

When we arrived at Room 204, Mits and I placed the luggage on the bed and looked around the room.

"A private room," I said expansively. "That's nice. Well, Mits, we've made it so far."

"Uh-huh," she said uncomfortably. "Shall we put your luggage away?"

Before I could answer, a familiar nurse appeared in the doorway.

"Darlene!" I hugged her gratefully, and we recalled the times we had gone through as patient-and-nurse in earlier surgeries. Post-operative procedures aren't always the most modestly-approached situations. Having a nurse with a lively sense of humor allows a patient to laugh at the ridiculous or bizarre.

After Darlene left I looked at the familiar hospital gown left by the nurses, opened my suitcase, and took out my robe and slippers I knew from past experience I would need to keep warm during my stay. With these I re-dressed for the occasion.

Next to my bed I arranged my reading and writing materials. Then, I placed two soft pillows I had brought from home at the head of the bed. I had just started to tape up cards and pictures on the wall to make it feel more like home when the phone rang.

"This is Arlene, from Dr. Dawson's office. I just wanted to call you to wish you good luck this morning with your operation."

"Why, thank you, Arlene," I said with surprise. At the doctor's office where I had seen her so many times in the past few years, Arlene was always cheerful, with a smile for each patient who filed past her desk each day. Her call made me think of the many people who had conveyed their best wishes to our family with calls and notes. I left out one note from my older brother to read again, and climbed back onto the bed.

Dearest Clo,

I believe God gives us life, and with it the opportunity to grow spiritually, and emotionally, as well as in stature...

You are a very special person, who I love and admire deeply...

You are a treasure to those around you. We hold you in our hearts, and in our hopes, and in our arms and harbor great hopes for you and your plans to write... for you and Glenn and your life together... for you and Moni and Bri, to watch them becoming two responsible people... for your rebirth of health and energy to share the treasures you hold within.

Lovingly your Bro,
Rob

I heard the sound of the gurney's wheels coming in the room. "Clo Hashiguchi?" the surgical nurse asked, checking my identification bracelet.

"Yes," I said, wanting suddenly to run for my life, far from this hospital. Why was I letting them take me into surgery again? This time it was not the same. They were not going to just fix something, so I would be better. There were no guarantees with this one. I may not even survive in the end. Lightheaded, I felt like I was floating in a surrealistic painting.

"How are you doing?" Darlene asked. She had come back and was sitting next to me on the bed, holding my hand, bringing me back to reality.

"Fine," I said, looking into her eyes. But that single word started an eruption of emotions. Deep sobs racked my chest. Darlene put her arms around me, allowing me to soak up her comfort as I laid my head on her shoulder.

"If you weren't a little upset by this, it wouldn't be normal, Clo," Darlene said quietly, allowing me to take my time. "It's okay."

"Thanks, Darlene," I said, struggling to gain control of myself. With every bit of courage I could muster, I forced myself to climb out of the bed, and onto the gurney. My body was cold and clammy, my stomach cramping in fear.

"You can wait with her, if you like," the surgical nurse said to Mits. "or I'll show you the waiting room." Off we went, down the corridor, through the surgery doors, rolling up behind another person awaiting her turn for surgery. Mits had opted not to go to the waiting room. She didn't have much stomach for what went on behind surgical doors.

When I had my first surgery two years ago, I waited there for three hours. I hoped this time it would go more quickly. I peered around me, observing the blue surgical masks, gowns, and booties on everyone around. It was like having arrived on another planet, listening to the padded feet shuffling all around me.

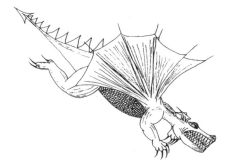

10

Mastectomy
I Made It!

A tall, thin man shuffled up alongside the gurney, identifying himself as my anesthesiologist for the surgery. After the usual questions, he said, "We'll give you sodium pentothal, so you will quickly go to sleep. We'll monitor your heart and respiration all the time you are asleep. You'll be well looked after." He stopped. "I can't guarantee there won't be any problems, but I'll do my best. I'll be there the whole time to try and keep you out of trouble."

"Thanks," I replied, trying to keep calm. I asked a nurse for another warm blanket. My body felt like ice. I could feel it shaking.

Dr. Dawson stopped by, holding my hand. "We've got to keep you living!" he said firmly, with the wonderful warm smile of a tall, lanky baseball kid. He had been in surgery with me before. Knowing he would be there again was a great comfort.

Dr. Lennard also stopped by to say hello before putting on his surgical blues. "You're going to be okay," he said smiling, trying to reassure me with a pat on the blanket, then walked through the door after Dr. Dawson.

By the time the nurse came to wheel me into surgery, I was relieved, thankful to be getting it over with. The anesthesiologist tried to insert the needle into the vein on the upper side of my hand, without success. Finally he inserted the IV into the crook of my elbow, as doctors and nurses readied themselves in the theater of operation.

What is this?" the anesthesiologist asked me, pointing to the simple black and white woven bracelet on my wrist.

"My daughter made it for me," I said quietly. I thought of how Monica had made many colorful friendship bracelets for herself over the past few months. It had been a great source of pleasure to her. When she heard I was going into the hospital again, she came to me with a full collection of bracelets strung along her arm.

"Choose any one you want, Mom," she said generously, extending her arm for me to see each one clearly.

"You sure you want me to have one of these?" I asked, touched by her gesture.

"Yes," she insisted, her eyes sparkling. "Which one do you want?"

I searched through the colorful bracelets, finally choosing a striking black and white weave. "I'd like this one."

"Okay!"

"Do you think it will go on over my hand? It's bigger than yours."

"Sure." She slid it up over the other bands and off, then pushed it over my hand with some effort, to encircle my wrist.

"Thank you, Moni," I said, giving her a hug. "I'll wear it when I go to the hospital. Every time I look at it, I'll think of you." She smiled happily, turning to go back outside to play.

"I don't think there's any harm in her wearing it," the anesthesiologist was saying to the nurse. I smiled to myself, feeling encircled by Moni's simple act of caring. The anesthetic had begun to take effect. Things started to get fuzzy…then nothing.

The room was spinning as I tried to open my eyes. After many attempts to get my bearings, I finally realized with great relief, *it's over!* A tingling sensation spread over me. The surgery was done. My first sure sign of it was the nausea I felt every time a pump of PCA Demerol flowed through the IV. My left arm was held in a blue and white sling. On my chest was a wide athletic band which held bandages in place.

I tried to feel any sensation in that area, wondering if I could feel that my left breast was missing. Nothing. I was thankful that I couldn't see the stark loss just yet, though I was curious to see the result.

A nurse switched my IV to PCA morphine, which calmed down the nausea. PCA is a method of dispensing an IV medication, which is set up so that a patient can control by the push of a button how much medication he receives. It has been proven that a patient normally uses less pain medication by this method of application.

I spent the afternoon trying to wake up, though I continued to be a sleepy patient.

"Hi, Mom!" Moni called to me across the room, as she led the procession of Glenn and Mits through the doorway. A big smile lit up her face as she handed me a big *Get Well* card to read.

"Hi, Moni!" I said sleepily, still muddling through the fog of the drugs. Mits and Glenn sauntered in behind Moni, greeting me from a distance as they patiently waited for Moni to have a moment with me first.

"Thank you, Moni," I said, enjoying her being so near. "What a great card!" She smiled happily. "It's so good to see you, honey." It felt awkward, not being able to reach out and give her a hug.

"How're you feeling, Mom?" Moni asked as I attempted to open the card with one arm on an IV and one in a sling.

"Just fine, honey. It's done. The surgery's over. Now, all I have to do is get well."

I looked over at Glenn and Mits, who were exchanging meaningful glances. "Hi, Gooch," I said, grinning through the fog at him. "I'd sure like one of your big, warm hugs." He made his way over to the bed, putting his arm around me and all attached paraphernalia.

Brian had stayed home. "Mom, I don't want to come see you in the hospital," he had explained quietly a few days before I left. "I don't want to see you with all those tubes and everything in you."

"That's just fine, Bri," I said, thinking back at how he had come right away the first time I'd gone to the hospital two years ago, but ever since had recoiled at the idea. It had been a shock to see me so incapacitated—not able to talk or act normally.

"I'll come maybe the second or third day, okay?" he asked. "It's not that I don't want to see you...It's just that..."

"It's okay. You don't have to come at all, if you don't want to, Brian," I said. "I'll miss seeing you, but I respect your feelings about this. I know you love me." I reached over, giving him a half-hug. "You've seen me in the hospital a lot—perhaps too much."

He looked down at his feet. "I don't want you to die, Mom," he said, almost in a whisper.

"I'm not going to die, Bri. I have so much to live for—you and Moni, and Dad. I have a very fine doctor who will be taking good care of me." I put my hand under his chin, lifting it up so I could look into his eyes, thinking how much I loved my children.

Since that first surgery, Brian had repeatedly discussed his fear of the possibility of my death. The impending surgery wasn't helping.

"This is going to turn out okay, Bri. I'm going to work very hard to get well. You're going to have a healthy mom again. After I get well...I'll race you!" I tousled his hair, grinning at him. "And I just might beat you!"

"Uh-unh!" he challenged, grinning back. Then: "I'll really miss you, Mom."

"You better practice your running!" I warned. "I'm going to get *good*!!" He got up off the bed, and sauntered out of room, smiling. I hoped I could pull it off.

We were all thankful the surgery had gone well. I was not aware of how terrified Mits was, still waiting for the test results to come back about the fourteen lymph nodes the doctor had removed. After surgery he had told her that we weren't home free until we had good results from those tests. She had lost her husband to cancer some years before, and she was scared.

As she and Glenn walked out the door with Moni, though, I could not see how heavy her heart was. She had only let me see her happiness that the surgery had gone well. All I knew was that I had survived having my breast removed, and the cancer with it. The surgery was completed, but the journey had just begun.

"I just thank God for a second chance to live."
— George Fawcett, breast cancer survivor

"The doctor said, 'Don't worry about it [a lump]. You're too young.'"
— Debbie Collier, breast cancer survivor

"I don't want to die."
— Tara Havemeyer, breast cancer warrior

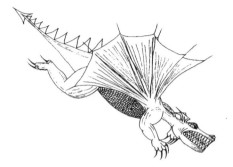

11

Visitors, Naps and Nausea

Reach to Recovery

My left hand in a sling, and right elbow restricted by the IV needle, I inched over to switch on the light. I reached for something humorous to read. It was early morning: darkness blanketed the sky. Stillness, occasionally peppered with a cry for a nurse, permeated the hallways. I shifted to try to find a comfortable position and opened the first book.

"Sometimes I get an almost irresistible urge…to go on living."

"There has been an alarming increase in number of things I know nothing about."

"Let's not complicate our relationship by trying to communicate with each other."

The book title seemed, under the circumstances, most appropriate of all: *I May Not Be Totally Perfect, But Parts Of Me Are Excellent,* by Ashleigh Brilliant.

After some time, I picked up one of my other favorites, *The Portable Curmudgeon*, by Jon Winoker:

"A cynic is not merely one who reads bitter lessons from the past, he is one who is prematurely disappointed in the future."

— Sidney Harris

"If all economists were laid end to end, they would not reach a conclusion."

— George Bernard Shaw

"Fashion is a form of ugliness so intolerable that we have to alter it every six months."

— Oscar Wilde

Absorbing the humor helped me to alter my bruised perspective, allowing me to take a lighter view of myself. Like stepping outside of this moment in time, I could observe things from a distance, a different angle. Like shedding skins, laughing helped me shed the old one, so that I could put on a fresh, new one.

The rest of the day was filled with visitors, brief naps to ward off the fatigue, and an off-and-on battle with nausea. Cards and colorful flowers continued to arrive, filling the room with warm wishes and sweet fragrance.

"Clo Hashiguchi?" A tall, slender woman in a stunning blue knit suit inquired, stepping confidently up to my bed.

"Uh-huh," I said sleepily.

"I'm Pat, from Reach to Recovery," she said cheerfully. The nurse had asked me the day before if I wanted one of the ladies from the American Cancer Society who had gone through a mastectomy before to pay me a visit. American *Cancer*...Society! I had said to myself, catching my breath, but aloud, I had replied, "Sure." Perhaps I could get some helpful advice on how to more effectively deal with the recovery, once the cancer was gone. I refuse to be a statistic, I stubbornly told myself.

She brought out a green cloth bag, out of which she pulled a small pink pillow and a hand-made prosthesis filled with pillow stuffing, to place where my breast had once been. She handed them both over carefully to me.

"We have volunteers who come and make all of these things for us," she informed me. "The volunteer men who were helping us enjoyed making the "boobs" *far* too much," she said with a twinkle in her eye, "so I have given them the small pillows to make, instead."

I chuckled, responding to her infectious laughter.

Trying to follow her stories through a medicated fog, I listened as Pat began to explain how she had joined Reach for Recovery.

"I had a bilateral," she said matter-of-factly.

"Both sides?" I said incredulously, looking at this very attractive, stylish woman through new eyes. I would never have guessed!

"Yes," she smiled. "One breast I lost because of cancer, and the other because they discovered numerous cysts in it through the years. It was also fibrocystic, plus there was a history of cancer in my family from my mom and dad. I decided it was better to *live* than to take a chance with the other breast, so I had them remove it, too."

"Did you have reconstruction?" I asked with interest.

"Yes," she answered, pushing in one of her breasts gently. "See!" she said, laughing. "It's soft, just like a normal breast would be. I'm really glad I had the surgery." She turned back to the small green bag, and began pulling out exercise gear, designed to hasten the recovery.

First, she brought out a bright red rubber ball, which she squeezed hard several times, explaining that this exercise would begin to bring back the hand's strength. Then, out came a long cord, with two wooden tongue depressors tied to either end. She looped it over the top of the door, demonstrating how to sit facing the edge of the door, pulling down on the rope with one hand, which would pull the other arm up, stretching the muscles of the injured arm. She explained that I should repeat it for the other arm, taking turns back and forth until I tired.

"It will take a while to be able to do it all the way," she said, "but just keep working on it. It will come."

She then showed me how to "walk" up the wall with the fingers of the injured arm.

"At first, you will only be able to go up a little ways," she explained, "but, if you work on it, you'll soon be able to 'walk' up until your arm is fully extended.

"These exercises will not be comfortable, but they will help bring back your arm's full range of motion." She demonstrated several other exercises, then told me: "Don't start any of these exercises until your doctor says you are ready, to prevent any injuries to the wound, okay? The doctors worry about that part of our visit, that maybe the patient will start doing the exercises without their authorization. So, we always try to say very clearly to wait for the doctor's instructions before you begin."

"That makes sense," I answered, trying to collect all of the words she had just shared with me.

"And," she said quietly, "it's okay to cry. I cried a lot. It hurts to work out those muscles. You'll get frustrated, but just keep working on it. It helps if you have people around you who care what has happened."

"I have a wonderful support system," I said through my haze. I felt my eyelids falling closed, in spite of all my efforts. I desperately wanted to sleep.

"If you have any questions at all," Pat said in leaving, "just give me a call. That's why I joined Reach for Recovery, to help others know they can get through it. If I did, you can, too!" Her radiant smile filled the room with hope.

"Thanks for coming," I said sleepily. All I could remember was that beautiful blue knit suit, and how normal she looked. She was actually laughing and joking, as if dealing with cancer were just as ordinary as dealing with the flu. It was a matter of working to regain my health. Nothing more, nothing less.

Dr. Lennard breezed in a bit later. "You did great!" he smiled. "Everything went well in surgery. We'll check to see how it's doing today."

He began by taking off the sling that held my left arm. He then removed the wide ace bandage, which held the dressings in place, applying pressure to the wound. Finally, he took the dressing itself off, piece by piece.

"Do you want to see how it looks?" he asked.

"Yes," I said with mounting curiosity.

"It looks good!" he said, obviously pleased with the results of his surgery the day before. I gazed down at my chest, struck by the simple lack of contour. The incision looked so unimposing, as though nothing of significance could have occurred there. Two flaps of skin stretched flat against my chest, held simply by steri-strips, not clamps as had been the case with my abdominal surgery. My eyes followed the zigzag wound winding purposefully across my chest to disappear under my armpit. He waited patiently as I scanned the results.

"It looks better than I thought it would," I said. "And, no stitches!"

"There are stitches inside," Dr. Lennard replied, "but we used steri-strips to hold the two flaps together on the outside so there would be less scarring after it heals."

"It looks like a beautiful job," I observed, impressed with how smooth the wound looked, and how cleanly it was held together with the careful stitching. "It helps to have a fine surgeon."

Carefully he removed the dressing from around the surgical tubings from the Jackson-Pratt drain. The two surgical tubings were stitched to the outside of two holes punched in the remaining skin below the armpit, to allow drainage of liquids and blood from the chest wound.

I winced, seeing the tubes hanging out from punched holes in my chest skin. Two flat rectangular drains had been attached to the tubing and inserted underneath the skin flaps during surgery to prevent a build-up of fluids in the wound as it began to heal. The surgery had been performed with the idea that in six months I would return for reconstruction. I was excited about the possibility and delighted at the doctor's workmanship.

"It's healing beautifully," the doctor said. "Let's check your range of motion." Taking my left wrist in his hand, he began rotating my arm to see how far it would go with comfort. "Tell me if it's uncomfortable," he said, as he worked it around.

He rotated it wider and wider. "This is great!" he said. "You only have about another 30 degrees to go, and you'll have it all back!"

Then he offered some warnings. "You must be careful the rest of your life of infections on this arm, because we have interrupted the normal flow between lymph cells. You should always wear a glove from now on when you work out in the garden. You don't want any dirt to get under your fingernails that could cause infection. If your fingers start to swell up, or your arm, that's what it is. Maybe you have seen older women with their arm swollen up, with an ace bandage wound around it?"

"Yes," I answered. "I guess I have," trying to remember clearly.

"They have what is called lymphomylitis" [lymphedema].

So, I have to wear a glove the rest of my life? I thought.

"And," he continued, "don't lift heavy objects with this arm."

A mental image of a limp, left arm emerged in my tired mind. "I'll do what I need to do to be well," I said matter-of-factly.

"We're still awaiting the lab reports," he said cautiously, his smile fading. "I'll let you know just as soon as they come back."

"Sounds good," I said, unworried. I felt like we were over the worst of it, and that the rest would turn out well. I did not realize how anxious the medical personnel and my family were for the results of those final tests.

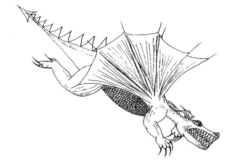

12

Negative Lymph Nodes

Choosing Against Chemotherapy

The next day, I was catching up with my journal when he walked in.

"Fourteen negative nodes!" crowed Dr. Dawson, as he promenaded into my room. He tweaked my toes that stuck up underneath the blanket, as if to emphasize the good news. "The nodes came back on the lab report *negative*. The rest of the lab report Dr. Lennard will talk to you about, but I just wanted you to know!" he said jubilantly. Obviously he was relieved, and very happy for me.

"Great," I responded, somewhat surprised at his relief. I had expected them to be negative, having been spared the stark reality of the high odds I was up against with such a large tumor. Nurses started to stop by to congratulate me. It dawned on me in my foggy state that if the nurses and doctor were that relieved, it was probably something that needed to be shared with my family.

Mits answered the phone at our house. "Cloey! How are you doing?"

"All the nodes came back negative," I told her simply.

"That's wonderful!" she responded. I heard her choke up on the other end of the phone. "That's wonderful, Cloey," she repeated. "I'm so happy!" I realized then just how worried she had been. She was not one to exhibit emotion.

A little while later, the phone rang.

"Hi, Sis."

"Hi, Rob. Thank you for the tree!"

"The tree?" my brother asked, puzzled.

"The poinsettia," I answered, laughing, enjoying his brief bewilderment. "It's huge!"

"What color is it?" he asked. He had wired the flowers.

"White with pink centers. It's beautiful!"

"Great!" he responded with satisfaction.

"And, thanks for the note," I added. "It was a real comfort."

"That's good. That's what I intended it to be."

"We need to check the JP drain," the nurse told me matter-of-factly after her usual cheerful greeting. She lifted the covers to do her inspection.

"It's draining well," the nurse commented as she opened the tubing to drain the bloody liquid discharge from my chest into the measuring cup.

"How much this time?" I asked, curious.

"Twenty milliliters," she answered, intent on her task.

I peered at my stitched skin. She had just changed the dressing, and was finishing up by emptying the Jackson-Pratt drain. Seeing those stitches once again, with tubes hanging through the punched-out holes, made me wince. I understood they were necessary, and was fascinated with the technique used to take care of the problem of chest drainage, but it still made me queasy. As the fluid drained out, I wondered if there were cancer cells flowing out, as well, and if there were any more left behind, not yet discovered.

She clamped off the tubing to prevent any leakage, noting on her chart the amount of liquid in the receptacle.

"Can I get you anything else?" she asked cheerfully, refilling my water cup.

"No, I think I'm fine. Thanks."

I was beginning to feel quite cocky about how *fine* I was feeling, using both restricted arms and remembering to tighten and flex my left hand at every opportunity, as my friend Georgia had earlier directed me to do. My head was clearing, but this afternoon I was feeling the need to stay quiet and reflect on what was happening, as well as what lay ahead.

Father, thank you for your care, and for the caring of all of the hospital staff as we walk through this.

A question entered my mind. "Do you really want to have chemotherapy?"

Do I *want* to have chemotherapy? I responded, taken aback by the question. I didn't know I had a choice.

The question persisted at length. I turned it over in my mind, exploring it from every angle, like a newly discovered jewel. Well, I suppose, if I could still get well and have the choice, I'd rather not. No, I guess I really don't want to have chemo. I really don't. No chemotherapy. I began to feel stronger and stronger about this new idea.

An overwhelming sense of peace rolled over me, as if the choice had then been made. Still meditating, I started to think about how I might be able to alter my diet to best support the healing of my body.

With all of the foods, additives, and chemicals believed to encourage cancerous growth, not eating at all seemed the safest route. However, since that choice seemed rather short-sighted in the end, I simply decided to eat the healthiest, most basic foods I could find, and hope for the best. Vitamins, minerals, and herbs might be able to fill in any gaps in my diet and offset other negative effects. I decided to pursue my best options when I arrived home.

Another idea, at first unwelcomed, came to mind. Ellie had a friend who was a psychic healer. The psychic healer's unusual abilities were significant enough to have been studied by a local university. Even then, she preferred to keep a low profile to prevent interruptions of her private life. So, why was I afraid to see this lady?

I wasn't anxious to make myself open to someone with unknown powers. I had grown cautious through the years of placing myself in a vulnerable position to another, realizing that others may not always have my best interests in mind. I finally decided that I would go if Ellie accompanied me, and would reserve the right never to return if I didn't want to. With that decision made, I felt at peace and drifted off to sleep.

I had learned with my previous surgeries that having something of Mom's from the hospital made my absence easier for my kids at home. When the family came to visit that evening, I offered the miniature pink pillow to Moni which Pat had left me. Her eyes sparkled happily as she accepted it.

"What's this, Mom?" asked Brian, holding up what he'd found on the windowsill.

"I thought you might be drawn to that, Bri," I chuckled. "It's the sling that they put on my left arm after surgery. Go ahead, you can have it. Try and figure out how it works." He fitted the sling across his chest, with a great, triumphant grin on his face.

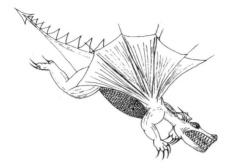

13

Coming Home

The Children's Reactions

The morning brought an unexpected visitor. I watched curiously as a teetery old gentleman found his way slowly, with difficulty, up to my bedside.

"I am a chaplain for the hospital here," he offered. "Jill—she's your sister-in-law?"

"Yes," I answered, still curious.

"She said that you might like a visit from me," he said simply.

"How nice," I said, touched by Jill's gesture.

"I can tell you're a loving person," he said as he stood beside my bed. "So is Jill. She gives me a hug every time she sees me."

After talking with me for a few moments he hesitated a bit, collecting his thoughts, then went on.

"My wife and I have been married 50 years. We just had our Golden Wedding Anniversary. We're so much in love; my wife says to me as I leave to come to the hospital, 'I can't wait till you get back. I'll miss you for the two or three hours you are gone.'" He grinned reflectively. He asked me a few more questions, then began to pray. His prayer was one of simplicity.

"Thank you for Clo and her loving family. Bless them as she goes through to recovery. Be with them. In Jesus' name. Amen."

My eyes glistened as he finished. There wasn't an insincere bone in his body. The energy surrounding him was like a window to the sun. As I watched him shuffle away, I was touched by his dedication to help those of us who were ill, in spite of his own fragile physical condition, and felt blessed.

The nurse soon arrived, instructing me carefully how to keep a record of the JP drainage, to be taken three or four times a day in milliliters. She provided me with four by four gauze pads, and paper tape for changing the dressing at the JP site daily.

"Watch your temperature," she cautioned. "If there is a change in your temperature or in the incision—increased swelling, drainage, redness, or increased pain— contact your doctor."

"Sounds fine," I said. All was well. I was going home. I had even managed to wash my hair by myself in the sink before breakfast. I felt great.

Soon Mits arrived, and together with the nurse, we carried suitcases and flowers out to the hospital entrance—me in a wheelchair, and Mits going ahead to get the car.

All the way home, I was aware of how wonderful it was to have the surgery over with and to be returning home.

"Mommy! Mommy! Mommy!" I heard my son chirping happily as the kids came bounding in the backdoor from school. Down the hallway their feet pounded. It was so good to hear the normal sound of my children's voices. Seeing them bounce in, faces aglow, was even better.

"Hi, Mom!" they both greeted me happily, giving me hugs.

"How are you feeling?" Brian asked, looking me over.

"Just fine," I said cheerfully. "It's so good to be home!"

Brian took off for the kitchen to search out a snack, while Moni lingered.

"Can I see it?" Moni asked me openly.

"No," I answered quickly, taken aback. "Not right now. Perhaps later." I didn't feel ready to expose my wound at the first greeting, and was concerned with the impact on her, being a young woman herself.

"*Please*, Mom," Moni said. It reminded me of what they had both spontaneously asked before I went into the hospital when I said there was a lump the doctors would be taking out.

"Can we see it?" they had asked eagerly. "Bring the lump home in a jar, so we can see it," they both begged. I just laughed out loud.

"I don't think so," I answered them, "but I'll see." The wonderful open curiosity of children is a delight. I could just imagine the doctor's reaction if I told him my kids wanted to take the tumor home in a jar to examine it. As it turned out, other things took precedence at the hospital. I never requested the tumor to be brought home.

Moni persisted.

"You really want to see it?" I asked her. Maybe she needed to see it. Maybe it would bother her more not to see it? She handled things quite differently than I at times. Perhaps now was one of those times.

"It doesn't look pretty, honey. It's healing beautifully, but it isn't very nice to look at." I looked carefully at my daughter, trying to decide what to do. I could see it was turning into a judgment call.

"I can *handle* it, Mom," she said, impatient at my warning.

"Okay," I said slowly, still with some hesitation. I carefully pulled back my housecoat to reveal the place where once a nicely rounded breast had been. The flattened area appeared stark; the long, scarlet diagonal wound fanning out across my chest, as Moni tried to take it in.

"Ugh!" she said with considerable feeling. I sensed that her reaction was more than she had anticipated. She just stared at the empty place. "It's gone!" she said with disbelief.

"Yes, but they're going to build me another one right where the old one was," I said softly, trying to ease the blow. She abruptly got up from the bed as I continued. "The doctor said it's healing beautifully..." I stopped. She had had enough. She walked briskly into the kitchen where her grandma was preparing dinner.

"They took off Mommy's boob!" she said quietly to her grandma.

"I know," Mits answered.

"It looks awful," continued Moni, having difficulty believing what she had just seen. Mits put her arm around her shoulders.

"But, they're going to make her another boob," Moni said, looking up hopefully.

"I know," Grandma responded. "Isn't that something! It's wonderful what the doctors can do now."

Over the next couple of days, I told each of the children I had had cancer, but that now I was healing, and would get well again.

The next day Brian asked to see the wound.

"Monica got to see it," Brian said forcefully. "If she could handle it, I can." So, I made the decision to take care of the detail with my son in the most respectful, calm way I could. First, I set it up by explaining the way the surgeon cut the skin, folded back the flaps, and took out the tumor and tissue. Then, how the drains were inserted—one on the top, and one on the bottom to insure the liquids would be removed, and healing would occur more quickly. Then, I explained that there were not clamps or stitches on the outside, just steri-strips visible from the outside to close the wound. Brian always liked to know how things worked.

"Are you sure you want to see it?" I asked again, remembering Moni's reaction the day before.

"Yes, Mom," he said decisively. "*Please.*"

I opened my robe to let the afternoon light from the window fall on my chest, feeling very exposed, but respecting the need each of my children seemed to have to deal with the realities of this situation. We had always been quite open with our children, respecting their need to know. However, this situation entered unknown territory. There were no easy answers.

"Ugh! It looks like it hurts!" he said with feeling.

"It is sore," I said matter-of-factly. I showed him where the drain tubes wove back and forth across the wound underneath the skin.

"If you touch here," I explained, "It's very tender because it rests against the wound inside. So, if you hug me, don't hug tight on that side."

"I can hug you on this side, then, right?" he asked as he demonstrated a small hug on my right side.

"Still gently, though, Bri. All right?"

"Okay," he said.

I explained how they would be reconstructing another breast for me.

"Will it be foam?" Brian asked, exploring future possibilities in his mind.

"It may well be," I answered. "It will be nice and soft, like the breast is naturally. So, it could be. I don't know."

He walked out of the room, down the hallway, and into the kitchen.

"Mom's gonna get a new boob," he said matter-of-factly to his grandmother.

In the months to follow, many "boob" jokes emerged as we struggled to deal with the daily realities of a one-breasted mother in the family. The word breast faded into the background, seeming too serious a reference to an already far-too-serious situation.

That night Brian strode into the bedroom, sitting down carefully next to me on the bed.

"I told Adam what happened, Mom," Brian said, waiting for my reaction.

"That's okay," I reassured him. "That's what friends are for—to share things that are important to us."

Silence. "Is it all right if I tell him about the cancer, Mom?" he asked softly.

"Yes, of course, Bri," I responded. "But, understand that I don't have it anymore. It's gone. I don't want you worrying about it, okay?"

"Travis's mom had cancer, didn't she, Mom?" he persisted. I could see the wheels were turning fast.

"Yes, honey," I said quietly.

"Didn't they find it in time?" he asked carefully.

"Probably not. It was a different kind of cancer, though," I explained. "There are lots of different kinds."

"Did she die of cancer, Mom?" he probed.

"Yes, she died of cancer," I answered him truthfully. My children had had to deal with the possibility of my death just months before when I had had to call 911 to help me breathe. I knew he was terribly worried about the outcome of this surgery. I took his head gently in my hands, and turned his face towards me.

"But I'm not going to die, Bri," I said as strongly as I could. "The cancer is all gone. We had an excellent surgeon, and many people who have been praying for us. I'm sure that has made a big difference. I have lots to live for. I am going to be working very hard to get well. I love you, Bri."

"I love you, too, Mom," he said hanging his head. "I just don't want you to die." he added with great feeling.

"I don't want to, either, Bri."

"I have a bad stomachache, Mom," Moni said in the morning.

"I'm not surprised, honey," I responded, "after the week we've had. All the decorations you put up to welcome me home, and the lemon meringue and apple pies you helped Grandma bake, the Rice Krispie bars you made, and all of the help you've given Grandma. You've been wonderful! I'm not surprised it's getting to you. You've put out a lot, Moni. I love you very much. Now, is there anything I can help *you* with?"

"I just don't feel good," she answered. But by the time she had showered and readied herself for school, there was no more mention of a stomachache. She threw on her pink cream-puff coat, gave me a quick kiss. Running down the stairs and out the door to catch the school bus, she called out cheerfully, "I love you all!"

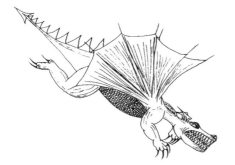

14

Constant Pain

Exhaustion

"Oh, no!" Mits groaned. "The funeral is Friday night? Where?" I lay on the bed, overhearing the brief plans made with her sister, Chiyo, on the phone.

"Do you think you'll be okay if I go to the funeral, Cloey?" Mits asked me.

"I'll be just fine," I smiled.

"I'll stay at Chiyo's, since the funeral is Friday night at the Buddhist church in Seattle. I have to get my hair done. It looks awful to go anywhere."

"You need a break from this, Mits," I said. "It will be good for you to get your hair done. It'll make you feel better. I'll just putter around here, catch up on my journal, and put on Christmas music and dance. That happy rhythm is good energy for me. It will help me get well."

"That's good," she answered, following up with a characteristic caution not to overdo. Then she reassured me: "All the laundry is done, and I'll make sure there's wood. I'll have Bri bring in a bucketful for you."

The next morning Mits built both fires hot, carried in the wood, and with Glenn, got the kids off to school. Wood was stacked three containers deep from the fireplace when she left, along with a glove for me to use, so my left hand would not get injured.

Hearing the door close, I padded to the stereo and put on some Christmas music. I danced back and forth a bit to the familiar sounds. Then it was time to collect the dressings for cleaning up the wound, the measuring container for drainage, my shampoo, a clean washcloth, and a large, fluffy towel.

I had been sponge bathing the best I could since I had come out of surgery. I missed that lovely flow of warm water. However, I did not want to risk any complications by wetting the dressing on my chest.

It was the first time I would face myself alone and naked since surgery. Survival had been the primary issue at the time of surgery—the physical impact of the loss of my breast hadn't fully filtered through my senses. I wanted to allow myself the time to do that this morning.

Unsnapping my housecoat, I gazed at the small dressing patched over the sutured holes, where drainage flowed out of the wound. Across my chest, the top and bottom flaps of skin lay flat, where once my breast had been.

I looked at my mangled body. The zigzag diagonal cut ran from nearly my breastbone all the way up into my left armpit. The surgeon was excellent. No stitches were showing at all. No clamps, only thick steri-strips holding this enormous incision closed from one end to the other.

I ran my fingers gently over the place where the two tubes protruded, encircling each other like snakes throughout the wound. At their points of departure from the body, black stitches had been firmly entrenched in the flesh to hold them in place.

That looks like it would hurt more than it does, I thought. I tried to sense any discomfort there, but could feel no pain.

How would this area look, inflated with a prosthesis? I wondered. And the nipple, would it look like my other one?

I emptied the JP drain, noting 45 cc of liquid on my tally sheet. After taping the dressings in place, I surveyed my masterpiece in the mirror, thinking: I've done it!

Finishing my sponge bath, I topped it off with some deodorant on my right side. Well, that's one good thing, I chuckled to myself. I'll save on deodorant, if I only need to put it on one side!

The next morning I arose at 5:30. Clumsily, I lit the upstairs and downstairs fires, using far more paper than any respectable Girl Scout to spark the fire. As my family slept, I puttered around the house, picking up a shoe here, and a cup there.

Before we knew Mits would be gone, arrangements had been made for each of the kids to have a friend over to visit in the afternoon. It would be a welcome diversion for them. I could see no reason why we should change our plans. It would probably be easier for me to watch the kids with one of their friends occupying their time, and Glenn would be home to help. He got up, made breakfast, and we assigned family jobs.

"What else do you need me to do?" Glenn asked me after we had eaten. "I can do laundry or anything else."

"Would you take Brian for a haircut?" I asked, sipping the hot green tea.

After lunch, the children's friends arrived. The father sat down to visit, asking how things were going.

"Fine," I said, enjoying the bit of conversation with another adult. We talked about our kids, about our families, then…

"I had Hodgkin's disease when I was younger—then melanoma two years ago," he offered. "It was a mole that changed color. So I know something about what you are going through."

Shocked, I thought how little we know about what goes on in people's lives around us. "I'm sorry. I didn't know you had cancer, Dave."

"I'm doing fine now, though I still get really tired at nights."

"I know what you mean."

In and out of the house, the kids' questions and the hustle and bustle of their excitement began to take its toll. I tried to lie down and rest as much as possible, but just the energy it took to answer a question became too much for me to handle. So I referred them outside to Glenn with their questions. Every so often Glenn came in to get a cold pop, asking if there was anything else he could do.

By late afternoon, I couldn't handle another question, even from Glenn.

That evening before dinner, Ellie and her husband, Eldon stopped over to deliver a Christmas wreath. Ellie took one look at me and said, "You're tired, Clo. I'm beginning to be able to read you too well."

"It's been a big day," I said tiredly, tears brimming.

We all sat down for a cup of tea. I was amazed how much better I began to feel after sharing a few minutes with good friends. Ellie secured a promise from Glenn that he would put the wreath up on the door for me, and they departed.

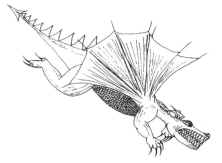

15

The Dressing, Tubes, Drain ...

Feeling Ugly

By dinnertime, Mits had arrived. I was lying down, trying to relax enough to be able to rest. I was beyond tired. Their cheerful chatter floated down the hallway. I waited until they were out of the kitchen, then found my way to the food to eat in quiet.

I couldn't handle being with anybody else. Just the possible stimulation of another person in the same room seemed overwhelming. I trudged slowly back to the bedroom.

Like water built up behind a dam, I felt tears of frustration ready to overflow. The frustrations of two weeks suddenly threatened to burst out.

"Gooch," I called decisively down the hallway. "Would you come here?"

I heard the familiar clump, clump, clump of his footsteps coming down the hallway.

"Gooch," I said, sitting up, trying to hold back the torrent of emotions, "I...I need you to help me handle what has happened." For days I had changed the dressing, routinely—even proudly—handling what was necessary, not realizing the deep well of feelings that were building up inside.

"I need you to *see* it, Gooch…and tell me you still love me." There, it was out, like a thorn taken from a wound.

He shrugged. "Okay," he said.

Slowly, I began to open my housecoat to my husband of 15 years, hesitating as tears ran down my cheeks. I thought of how my children had been repulsed. I couldn't see that duplicated in his eyes.

"It's all right, Willie," he said encouragingly.

"Tell me you love me," I said fearfully, searching his eyes.

"I love you, Willie," he said reassuringly.

Devastated, I turned my head to the wall, and opened the robe fully to his view, sobbing as I waited painfully for his reaction.

"I love you, Willie…" he repeated quietly. I turned back to look at him. No shock was reflected in his eyes, just kindness. His strong arms hugged me protectively, allowing me to regain my inner balance.

"Gooch," I explained after the tears subsided, "I need you to be at the helm when I'm recovering. I have so little energy. I need to spend what energies I have on getting well, or I don't think I'll make it."

"Also," I went on, leaning against the counter, "I've decided not to take chemotherapy. The doc says there's limited research supporting the recommendation of chemo in cases such as mine. I think my odds may be better if I take the hormone treatment, use visualization, watch my diet, exercise, and have a healer help me."

Glenn looked at me skeptically.

"Ellie has a friend who is a healer," I told him. "I'd like to check her out. I'll be able to tell if she's legitimate or not. You know that I have some abilities of my own in that area. If I don't feel comfortable with her, I will not go back. But, if things seem right, she may be able to help me regain my health again more quickly, if I combine it with hormone treatment rather than go through chemo. Chemo destroys good cells along with the bad. I don't think my body can take that now."

Glenn gazed silently at the floor as I spoke.

"But," I went on, "I need to feel your support. Will you back me?" I was aware that I was asking a lot.

He looked me over, shifting his weight to the other foot.

"I consider that stuff witchcraft...I'll really have to do some soul-searching on this one," he said carefully. "I don't want...to lose you," he said almost in a whisper.

"What about if we try it for a while to see if it works?" I inquired.

"Maybe we could do that," he responded.

Dr. Lennard had said Glenn and I would need some time alone to sort things out. In my mind I had pooh-poohed the idea, but later I was struck with how accurate he had been. Ultimately, the mastectomy was something we needed to deal with together. We had taken the first step.

Spent, I walked into the living room.

As I sat on the couch, my body, already in a state of fatigue, began reacting to the degree of stress I had just experienced, echoing the emotional upheaval with an unbearable muscle tightening over the entire area affected by the surgery a few days before.

For the first time, I became aware of severe pain in my left arm, and a numbness down the back of my arm from the shoulder to the elbow. It began to throb. Trying to think clearly through the pain, I decided that the tubes of the JP drain must have shifted upward inside the wound from the sudden and massive muscle constriction of the muscle tissue under duress. I was not knowledgeable regarding the anatomy of nerve cells enough to know if the tubes laid on them long enough whether they might produce permanent damage or not, but I was suspicious.

The skin across my chest got tighter and tighter...the pain was excruciating...I wanted to scream. I held my arm out to the side in an effort to alleviate the throbbing.

"Get it! Get it!" Moni yelled in excitement to her dad, as they played a computer game in Brian's room.

"*There*, not there!" she coached emphatically.

Brian snuggled up next to me on the couch, putting his arm around my shoulder, seeming to sense my pain. I said nothing. I thought I might lose it if I spoke.

Maybe the doctor should take out the tubes tonight if they are injuring something, I thought. I cringed at the thought of anyone touching the area. Just as I decided to call the doctor, my body began to relax, without explanation. The pain began to subside, becoming more and more bearable. I looked at my watch—9:30 p.m. Nine and ten o'clock were the visualization and meditation times set aside for me by my friends and family. Within fifteen minutes I was so relaxed that I gave a big yawn, and headed for the bedroom. I never mentioned the crisis out loud, but was extremely thankful it was over.

The next day, I mentally calculated and recalculated when I could take another Motrin for pain, and just how many hours I had before I could go into the doctor's office to get the JP drain removed. The pain was not as severe as it had been the night before but continued steadily, like a night train clicking persistently down the tracks.

Mits took the kids to a movie that day, so Gooch put on his shoes and I my blanket, and out the door we trudged for a ride in the country.

We wound along the narrow country roads. Down a long hill into the Snohomish Valley, the expansive greens and browns of the farms welcoming our weariness. The sharp peaks of the Cascade Mountains showed off the first snow-dusting of the winter cold in the distance.

"Look! Parachutes!" Across the valley two bodies were floating effortlessly down through the clear winter air to the cropland below.

"Look at the shape of the parachutes. They're rectangular!" I said in my excitement.

"That's the new design for parachutes," Glenn explained. "It minimizes the jarring of the body when the chute opens, plus it adds to the maneuverability."

The last figure down landed perfectly on his feet and walked a few feet forward to maintain his balance as the colorful parachute crumbled down beside him.

On the return, we decided to pool our pennies for two butter-scotch ice cream sundaes at the local Dairy Queen. I spooned into the rich sauce dribbling over the mountain of ice cream, each bite arousing memories of when Glenn and I were going together, and the first two butterscotch sundaes we ordered one hot, humid summer day near Kampsville, Illinois.

"People really seem to need you to be a hero. It's like you're under an obligation to do something miraculous."

— Patricia Van Kirk, breast cancer survivor

"We have suffered many losses—control of our lives, jobs, friends, sleep, marriages, finances, insurance, breasts, and often our hair. Hair loss for many is more traumatic than losing a breast and is obviously more noticeable."

— Linda Fankhauser, breast cancer survivor

"Hang in there!"

— Marie McClintock, breast cancer warrior

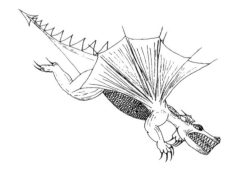

16

Excruciating Pain

Trying to Convince a Doctor It Hurts!

"You want some soup?" Mits asked each of us as we sat down to a hearty dinner of teriyaki chicken, rice, vegetables, and Japanese soup. "It has miso in it. It's good for you." I looked at the light brown broth, filled with napa and Japanese mushrooms. Mits had cooked this for the family's health, according to Japanese tradition. How she managed these extra touches was more than I could grasp. She had amazing energy.

As we all sat down to relax and watch TV after dinner, Gooch and I shared a glance and chuckled. No sooner had Mits sat down in the easy chair when she fell sound asleep.

"That was a good movie," Mits said later.

"How could you know?" we kidded her. "Your eyes were closed!"

"I could still hear it!" she protested, cocking her head and laughing.

The kids tucked into bed, I made my way painfully back to bed. By now I was constantly holding my arm out to my side at a 90 degree angle to relieve the pain from the JP drain. Tomorrow this will come out, I told myself. Not long now. I lay down on the bed, trying without success to find a comfortable position. The pain was worsening.

"How are you doing, Cloey?" I heard Mits ask through the pain.

"God, it hurts!" I said. "It doesn't ease up." My whole left side throbbed. My arm was arched across the left side of the pillow, like the arm of a discarded scarecrow. I was trying with all my will to relax enough to manage the excruciating pain under my armpit.

"Call Dr. Lennard," I said. "He told me to call if there was any change. This is definitely a change. It might be damaging something."

Mits scurried into the kitchen to find the phone number. By now my entire body was shaking uncontrollably, and suddenly, I became very cold. As I got up to get ready to go, I glanced at myself in the mirror. My face was ashen. My light brown hair looked nearly black by comparison against my colorless face.

"I don't know how many ccs," Mits was saying to the on-call doctor. "Just a minute. I'll ask her. Cloey, the on-call doctor wants to know how many ccs you got today."

"I'll talk to him," I said in desperation. I remembered I had not emptied the drain for a few hours. Maybe it wouldn't be enough...What was he looking for? Mits handed me the receiver.

"Doctor, the tube from the JP drain feels like it has shifted position. It is pushing up into the place under my arm where the nodes were taken out. The pain is excruciating. Can you take the tube out? I can't stand the pain anymore."

Silence.

"When did you have your surgery?" he asked matter-of-factly.

"Last Monday," I replied. "Can you help me? This is so painful!"

"How many ccs are coming out a day?" he asked.

"Just a minute," I answered, "I haven't measured the last of it today." In absolute agony, I called out, "Please help me!" Mits was right beside me as we made our way into the bathroom to measure the remaining liquid still inside the JP drain.

This man has not even acknowledged my pain, I thought to myself. All he wants to know is how many ccs of bloody fluid are coming out of my body.

Mits walked back and relayed to him, "30 ccs."

"Wait a minute," I said in a panic. Maybe if the figures weren't the right ones he was looking for, he wouldn't help me. "I'll talk to him." I began reading the log of figures I had kept for the past few days.

"It was 30 ccs tonight, which I was going to take in the morning. Can you help me?"

Silence. "30 ccs?" he repeated. "How many tubes are coming out of the drain?"

"Two," I said painfully. "This pain is EXCRUCIATING! Can you take it out? It's pushing into my armpit!"

Silence.

"IT HURTS LIKE HELL!" I finally cried out in agony. Maybe he didn't believe me.

"Where is the tube located?" he asked matter-of-factly.

"On the top," I answered. Was I talking with a computer? Barely able to control my frustration, I continued, "There is another on the bottom."

No response.

I was incensed by his repeated silence, and lack of responsiveness to my pleas for help for the pain. I wanted to scream at him over the phone; but I was afraid he would think I was just an hysterical woman, and my pleas for help then would be totally dismissed.

"Can you take it out?" I asked, fighting with everything I had to maintain control.

"Yes…you can come in to the hospital, to Emergency."

"I'll be there in 20 minutes," I replied immediately. "Will I meet you there?" I inquired.

"No, they can handle taking it out there," he said briefly. "I'll call this in to them."

My whole body relaxed a bit with the knowledge that I was going to get some relief. The pain seemed to subside somewhat, as Mits finished helping me get ready.

Gooch stood in the doorway. "I'll go warm up the car," he said quietly. I heard his familiar footsteps plodding down the hallway, down the stairway, and out the door.

~   ~   ~

"Do you like my outfit?" I quipped to Dr. Lennard the following day as he entered the examination room. "I dressed for the occasion!" I sat in my emerald green bathrobe, pastel striped dressing gown, and gray coat, with white slippers and long navy blue socks to keep my feet warm.

"I like your style" he said, chuckling. "How are you doing?" he asked.

"I took a trip to emergency last night to have one of the JP drains taken out," I relayed briefly. "The drain had shifted up into my armpit where the lymph nodes had been removed. The pain became unbearable."

"Ooh," he said, understanding the discomfort that must have caused. "How many ccs?"

"Oh! I forgot to bring the stats," I replied. "But I kept a record. I can tell you...37 ccs yesterday to 30 last night, plus what is left here today." A small amount of opaque red liquid sloshed back and forth inside the holding container.

"I'm sure it's fine," he said decisively. "Let's pull it." He carefully snipped the stitches attaching the tube to my skin.

I was amazed again, as I had been the night before in emergency, at the length of the surgical tube—about two feet long—being pulled out of my body. Then came the small, rectangular drain.

"It's out," he said with finality. "Oh-oh. It dropped some blood on your gown. I know blood can stain," he said to me as he worked the wet towel over the area, trying to get it out. "I'm sorry, it's wet now."

"That's fine," I said. "I'm just relieved to have the drain out. That'll wash out."

"The tumor board hasn't met yet, but I'd like to recommend hormone treatment—the tumor was so large," he explained. I was delighted. The last time we discussed it, he was talking chemotherapy. "If we go long-term, I'll talk to you about the side effects later. I'll be recommending hormone treatment, plus telling them about your style!" His eyes twinkled.

"Well, here," I lifted my leg to show him. "Would you like to bring one of my blue socks along to show them?" His sense of humor delighted me.

"Doc," I said reflectively. "I have to tell you about what happened last night." He turned around, walking back to the examining table where I sat. I told him about my experience with the unresponsive doctor on call.

"There was no acknowledgment of the pain at all," I said quietly. "That's why I called him, because of the pain. I told him again and again how bad the pain was, but the only response was silence and questions about the drainage. I wanted to scream at him into the phone." Tears were filling my eyes as the experience came back.

"If he could have just said, 'That must hurt.' It would have been enough. I never told him any of my other symptoms, because he seemed only interested in the measurement of the ccs. If it had been an older person with a heart condition, the results could have been disastrous, not getting the whole picture."

"I'm so sorry this happened," he said, taking off his glasses.

"I'm sure he's a very caring person, Doc," I said. "I've heard very fine things about him."

"I'm sure he was sitting there trying to figure out what to do," he said in explanation, "but that's too bad. I'm sorry you had to go through this."

"It was very dehumanizing," I said quietly. "Maybe you could let him know in a kind way, so that no one else will have to go through that again?"

"I will talk with him," he said kindly.

"Maybe he could do surgery on frogs!" I said suddenly. "Then he wouldn't have to talk!"

He laughed out loud. "Are you a frog?" he quipped.

"Not the last time I checked," I answered, laughing back.

"Sometimes I come in in the morning [for radiation]. The nurse asks me to step on the scale. I say, 'No.' She says, 'We need to get your weight.' I say, 'Not today.' They've gotten used to me. It's *my* body. Some days I don't want to be weighed."

> — Kathryn Gunther, breast cancer survivor

"I had this perception that women with breast cancer were dying. I see them now as loving and experiencing life. I'm so much more alive and aware of things, not taking life for granted."

> — Teresa Martinez, breast cancer survivor

"Somewhere, I've lost my dread and fear of death. I feel at peace. This is one good outcome of cancer for me."

> — Sharon Harnden, breast cancer survivor

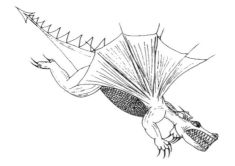

17

Simple Fact of Friendship
Therapy Works

"We are the injured body.
Let us not desert one another."
— Tillie Olsen, *Silences*

"Clo?" Jane said on the phone. "We'd like to bring you dinners for the next week. Would that be all right? The teachers and I really want to do this."

"But, Jane," I said, thinking of their schedules, "how can you do this? You all have such busy lives yourselves."

"We want to," she countered. "We thought it might help Mitzie out, too."

"It would be wonderful for Mits. It would help her a lot," I agreed, thinking of the enormous effort she was making each day.

"Good!" she said happily, and from that night the food started flowing in. By the end of the week we had so much food in the house we were floating in abundance. And, Mitzie hadn't had to make dinner all week.

In the weeks that followed, friends dropped by with food, gifts, and words of hope, but most important was the simple fact of their friendship and the faith that we could somehow find our way out of this jungle.

Some things went on as normal: Glenn dropped off Christmas calendars and fortune cookies for his customers; tantalizing packages began appearing under the Christmas tree; and the kids began singing the familiar Christmas carols. I don't think I ever understood just how beautiful those carols were before.

Being an optimist by nature, I assumed the worst was over. The drains out, I looked forward to a few exercises a day to strengthen my arm. It might be a little uncomfortable, but with the cancer gone —I was nearly done, I thought happily!

My friend Georgia had advised me to start moving the fingers of my injured arm as soon as I came out of surgery, to begin the strengthening process. Religiously, I followed her advice. I wanted to get well QUICK!

I was now a week-and-a-half out of surgery. Still on Motrin for pain every four hours, I was handling the nerve damage across my chest from the shifting of the JP drain quite well, though I was still a clock-watcher. Without the pill, it felt like a hot iron was being placed on my chest. With the pill, it was quite manageable most of the time.

Then it hit. Suddenly the wound's healing began to accelerate, and with it a rapid restriction of the skin flaps. Range of Motion took on new meaning, as I could barely rotate my arm.

Seeking relief, I stood in the shower, water as hot as I could stand it. Ahhh…hh! The warmth began to send relaxation through my entire body. Even though my whole side still burned from the nerve damage, it was not hurt by the flow of hot water.

Encouraged by the effect, I tried to rotate my left arm and shoulder back and forth in winged motion, elbow bent. I could feel the tight pulling under my arm, and across my chest. I was thankful I had just taken a Motrin. I extended my arm outward and upward as far as possible. One, two, three, four, five…nine, ten. I held my arm out in the farthest extension possible for the ten counts, just like I did for stretching exercises, then allowed my arm to relax, while I counted to ten as the hot water flowed over the working area. Again I stretched out my arm, and again allowed the hot water to relax the stretched muscles.

Walking my fingers a bit up the wall of the shower stall, I was amazed at how, even a few days before, this exercise would not have been the agony it was proving to be at this moment. Using the same technique, I allowed the water to relax the muscles between each determined attempt. Three times was plenty.

So, this is what they've been talking about—the exercises. Echoes of their warnings came back in my mind.

"They're rough, but you need to keep working through them," Dr. Lennard had advised. "Maybe it will take two to three months."

"It's okay to cry," Pat from Reach to Recovery had affirmed. "We all need to at times. It *hurts*! It took me four to five weeks each time to work through the exercises until I had recovered my range of motion."

"Good job!" I would say, talking my arm through its exercises. (I'm glad no one could hear me!) "I know it's hard, but we're going to make it." At times, I felt a little silly talking to my arms and chest as they progressed through the stages of healing, but an interesting thing happened as I began this dialogue: the sense of a partnership evolved. We were in this together, and each had an important part to play in achieving that goal.

"Learning to live with breast cancer is like inviting The Monster to tea!"

— Nikki Nordstrom, R.N.

"Working with breast cancer patients has been challenging and rewarding, but offset at times with sad disappointment when we fail."

— Dr. Stan Lennard, breast cancer surgeon

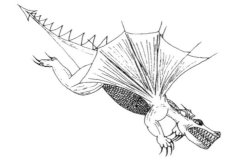

18

Meeting the
Oncologist

Depression Lifts

"I never felt fragile before. I've felt depressed, angry, joyful, sad,
hopeful, and excited, but never fragile. Having cancer has made me
feel like the petals of a rose, afraid of bruising, afraid that tomorrow
the frost will come, and my bloom will have passed with the thawing
of the ice crystals."

— Clo Wilson-Hashiguchi

January 12. I feel like a black hole caving in on itself. Why
can't I shake off this cloud of dark depression?

Only two weeks ago, Christmas was such a bright, joyful day,
the family celebrating around three live fir trees in the living room. The
trees were just saplings, but they proudly held as many ornaments and
bright lights as their wobbly branches could muster.

Now…sheer exhaustion…at nine o'clock in the morning. I'll
just tell the receptionist I'm not up to being here this morning so that I
can go home and get some sleep.

"Clo?" The nurse beckoned me into one of the cubicles, white,
with a doctor's examining table in the middle. Another doctor, I sighed.

"Just hear him out, Clo," Dr. Lennard had said when he mentioned that Dr. Sargur may ask if I wanted to be a part of a chemotherapy study.

"I'm not interested, but okay," I responded. "I'll hear him out."

Why are there so many of us women having mastectomies? I asked myself as I settled into the available chair, suddenly quite angry. One in every ten* women. It's far too many. Why is this happening to us?

Dr. Sargur came bustling in, books piled up under one arm, a notebook and charts in the other.

"Sorry I'm late," he said breathlessly. "I was picking up your files from Dr. Lennard's office."

"That's okay," I said, amused at his manner of entry.

He reached for a chair, rolling it over until it was directly opposite me. He sat down decisively, his intense, jet-black eyes lively, and focused on the moment—NOW.

"I'm Doctor Sargur," he said with friendly directness, "and you are Clo. I expected to see an Oriental, but Dr. Lennard told me you were Caucasian in every way," he said, grinning.

"Yes I am," I chuckled, enjoying his good humor.

"Can you tell me what you understand has happened so far in your case?" he asked, a distinct East Indian accent peppering his English.

"Two weeks before Thanksgiving I went in for a post-op exam for last year's operation in February," I began. "I felt a mass in my left breast, so had Dr. Asmussen examine me." Briefly, I reviewed my medical history over the past one-and-a-half months for him.

After listening intently, he said, "I have been following your case through Dr. Lennard, making recommendations to him as he came to me asking questions. Your tumor was large, but with the lymph nodes free—well, we'll see after we look over things today what we decide."

He began a detailed history of cancer of the breast and mastectomies, describing the treatments at each point in time, and in each appropriate country.

"Currently, in Europe when a lump is found," he explained, "a lumpectomy is usually done—just taking out the lump, and leaving the breast intact—followed by radiation. In the United States, the whole breast is usually removed—a modified radical mastectomy, which is what you had,** and then radiation, chemotherapy, or other adjunct therapy to follow, depending on the diagnosis. There is no significant statistical difference in survival rates between those patients who have simply had the lump removed, plus radiation, and those who have had the entire breast removed, with treatment. There are a lot of questions concerning this right now here in the United States. Which is better for the patient?"

He waited patiently while I pondered this new information, then asked, "How have your relationships been at home? Are you getting good support?"

"My family has been wonderful," I answered. "I have a great network of support."

"Good," he said. "A study of mastectomy patients shows that there are no significant changes in their relationships, unless they were unstable to begin with."

"Interesting," I said.

"The only long-term social effect of having a mastectomy, they have found, seems to be that the woman does not want to undress in public—like at the pool, or working out with others," he offered, studying my reaction.

"I felt that way," I said simply. It had taken me several weeks at the pool to be able to deal with the public exposure. I didn't expect it to bother me, but it did. After several heart-felt exchanges with other women with long-term illnesses, I felt free to take my shower openly. Now though, I sometimes felt an odd pang at the sideways glances I received as someone would suddenly notice the large red scar that slanted across where my left breast once lay. Unexpectedly, I would feel a poignant sense of loss, a sort of loss of innocence, as I watched the young women—their bodies whole—shower and dress, unaware of their wealth.

Dr. Sargur painstakingly continued my mastectomy education, making good use of the books he had carried in, pointing out specifics as he went along. I was impressed with how much time he was taking. He guided me through the information in my files, including the results of tests taken.

Like a college professor sharing significant research, he walked me through the many facts and explanations for nearly 45 minutes. I became keenly aware that he was not only sharing information he felt was important for me to know, but that research in the area of mastectomies was in its infancy. There were far more unknowns than knowns, far more questions than answers. It was in this gray area that he was challenging me to be a part of the decision-making process concerning my health and future, respectful of the part I would have to play in my recovery. I noted his dark eyes, reddened with overwork.

"How do you deal with all of this information?" I asked.

"We are dealing with too much information coming at us at a time to be able to sort it all out and process it on a daily basis for our patients. It's impossible to read it all. There are many new medicines coming out, but with new risks. Then it is our job to interpret it to each individual patient who comes in with a particular kind of cancer."

"That must be tough," I sympathized. "It must also be difficult to recommend a treatment to a patient, when everything is in its infancy—when there's so much gray area."

"That's right," he said candidly.

"Perhaps not all patients want to handle all of the information?" He nodded.

"I remember at one point all I wanted was a cure," I continued. "I was desperate. If Don Quixote had come in with an invitation to join him, I would have hit out at windmills gladly, if I thought it would have helped. There is such a feeling of vulnerability and desperation.

"I think it could be said that, as cancer patients, we all want a cure, and at some moments that is all we want. But even more important than offering us a cure is your respect and willingness to walk with us, a sort of guide through the rough spots, to help us handle this time with grace. It continues to amaze me how much it helps just to know someone else cares. It seems to allow my mind to give up part of its burden, and relax just a little, which enables my body to use more of its energy for the business of getting well, rather than worry."

"I appreciate you sharing this with me," he responded. "It helps me understand more how to help my other cancer patients."

"How do you deal with this every day?" I asked him.

"I like to help people," he said simply. He sat quietly for a moment. "It makes me think of my own mortality...and makes me appreciate my good health every day." Our eyes met in understanding.

"Clo, you are doing very well. There are people who are much worse. These people—their daily struggles are...are having to deal with how to handle the daily nausea, the daily pain." It was obvious how this touched him.

"You should visit the support group offered for cancer patients here, and see for yourself how lucky you are, how well you are doing, how little you have to deal with compared to some of them."

"Okay. It will give me a broader perspective of what is going on. I think you're right. It would be beneficial."

"There is a long-term study going on right now for those in your gray area. You can choose to be a part of that study, if you want. You can be in the group that takes tamoxifen, which does not kill the cancer cells which may be lurking around, but which stops more cancer cells from growing. Or you could be in the group that takes chemotherapy, which would kill the cancer cells that might still be in your body." Silence. "What would you like to do?" He stopped to look at me, waiting respectfully for my reply.

"The hormone treatment," I answered decisively. "No chemotherapy. I have taught creative visualization for some years," I added by way of explanation, "Some friends and I have been working hard on *visualizing* me well, in addition to the prayers lifted. No pie in the sky. It's hard work. We have had some incredible experiences with this thing, but I never questioned the ability of it to work."

"This is very interesting," he answered. "I have done some work on this when I was at the university. I took 15 students and did a study where we fed them CO_2 and told them it was O_2. In every case the mind/body compensated for the CO_2 by barely reacting to the straight CO_2.

I nodded. "I need to be gentle with my body to help it regain its health. Chemotherapy seems too invasive, particularly since it kills good cells as well as bad cells."

"Well," he answered, "hormone just *blocks* the cancer cell. It does not kill it. The chemotherapy *kills* the cancer cells."

"I know," I answered, accepting his assessment somewhat reluctantly. "There are no guarantees."

"After two to five years when we take you off the hormone treatment, we do it gingerly, not knowing exactly what will happen," he explained.

"It could be that there is no more cancer."

"Not necessarily," he said.

"Yes, but it *could* be," I said assertively, thinking: That's what I'm *counting* on!

*Today it is 1 in 8 women.
**An increased number of lumpectomies is being done in the U.S. today.

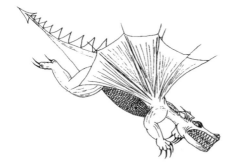

19

Helping Others with Cancer

A New Need for Privacy

"I can't hold anything down," Priscilla whispered on the other end of the phone. "Except a bit of popsicle today. I told my husband I felt so crappy everywhere that I just wanted to die."

"That must have been hard for your husband to hear," I responded. "How did he handle it?"

"I don't know," she answered. "But it was the truth." Priscilla is a vivacious high school secretary in her forties.

"How much chemo are you going to have?" I asked.

"Six months," she said. "Then two to three months of radiation. Did you have to have chemotherapy?"

"I had a choice," I replied. "I'm in the gray area, so I'm on tamoxifen. They don't really know…"

"How is your husband handling it?" she asked.

"He's been a wonderful support. Do you have friends you can call when you get really down, just to talk?"

"Yes, I do," she answered. "I can tell them just how I feel. They're great."

"Well, if it gets too much for them, feel free to call me. I've been down that black hole many times. There's nothing like it, is there?"

"No," she answered. She was still for a moment. "I have some friends who get angry with me. They wonder why I say such things. They say to be strong. They don't understand how I can talk about not fighting."

"They've never been there," I said simply. "If they had been dealing with this thing, they'd know."

"That's right," she replied.

"I have had to become very selective about who I spend time with. Some people can't handle what's happening. That's okay. But I don't have the strength to build them up, too."

Priscilla agreed. "A lady who was a cancer patient offered to talk with other cancer patients through the doctor's office. The nurse gave me this lady's name. We talked about an hour. Afterwards, I just sat down and cried for about half an hour. I was so depressed."

"Uh-oh," I said. "Stay away from her. Did you tell the nurse?"

"Uh-huh. She felt really bad."

"It's important she knows," I told her. "Do you meditate?"

"Not really," she answered. "When I get really down, I have books I read that help me keep my perspective. This is heavy duty. It's so tough not to lose it."

"Have you heard about the book called *We the Victors*?" I asked. "It tells about a number of cancer patients in New York. The author interviewed selected patients who had recovered."

"Sounds good."

"It is," I responded. "There was an interesting pattern through-out: each patient had at least one other person who helped him believe he could make it. We are fortunate to have good support systems. I don't know how people make it without one. Even having just one supportive person swung the balance in that book. It would be really tough on that one person, though. It's such an incredible thing to deal with."

"That's right," she said. "You're so easy to talk with."

"So are you."

"Thanks."

"We're going to make it, aren't we Priscilla?" I said with determination.

"Yes," she answered.

Before having cancer, I didn't realize it took so much energy to be around people. I've always sought out people of all kinds, to listen to their ideas. I feel privileged to hear their stories. This easy exchange of energy I had taken for granted. Now, abruptly, I was seeking out alone time as I had never done before. A feeling of detachment accompanied this tendency, as if I were watching a movie rather than being a part of the action. I sought out my plants, and in quietness tended to their needs, appreciating their beauty and simplicity.

One of my regular jobs that has evolved to maintain my inner balance is to get rid of that buildup of negative thoughts and fears that seems to store up in my mind. The process I've dubbed, *taking out the garbage.* I have observed that if I diffuse the buildup regularly, rather like cleaning house, I am able to better maintain that inner balance.

Getting rid of the *garbage.* I have found that what works for me is doing things that make me contented—like dancing, listening to music, creating a piece of art, reading, meditating, taking a walk, swimming, singing, laughing, spending time with a friend, or writing. Writing has been particularly helpful. Like sketching, it seems to pull out the inner tension, cord by cord, while sharpening my mental clarity and balancing my emotional well-being. Even physically, I feel better after my regular writing sessions.

"What are the emotions you go through in dealing with cancer?" Dr. Sargur asked me one morning. It would help me to know."

How can I tell him that, as a cancer patient, I try to show him my best side—so that the prognosis may somehow be affected in a positive manner, and therefore, offer me more hope. If he loses hope, it strikes my hope a mortal blow.

I've seen the look of futility in people who discover I have had cancer—looking for signs of my possible demise—at the same time offering me empty phrases of masked hope. Already they see me in my grave, my headstone mounted firmly above the mound of earth that covers my remains. Part of my personal battle as a patient is to keep that look of futility at bay in the eyes of those I meet. I want so desperately to believe I can beat cancer. Somehow, if others can see improvement, the odds appear to increase in my favor.

What the doctors do not see is the solo battle with fear and terror. It is an internal battle, one that is fought in all the hours of awareness, whether awake or asleep. On the way to work, in the middle of making pancakes or reading a story to a child, cold fear suddenly grabs hold of the heart and squeezes out all life and hope. Over and over, the cancer patient must fill that void. It's like being kicked over a precipice into a deep pit, with no handholds available.

"Now what?" the patient asks himself. "How do I get out? Hello!? Can anybody help me?" Then, "Is it *possible* for me to get out?"

When I cry out from those depths, it is as if the whole universe echoes with its sound. The journey up from the pit is an incredibly difficult effort. People ask why cancer patients give up. My astonishment comes from knowing so many keep on fighting to live.

I have described cancer as a dragon. Our challenge as cancer patients is to find the soft spot in the side of the dragon—to slay the dragon, then be done with him.

My emotions? The minute breast cancer was confirmed, my emotions went on a wild roller-coaster ride. The decisions we patients must make are made in the middle of that wild ride.

At times, the most difficult part is just to hold ourselves together in one piece—to wave good-bye to our children as they go off to school, to answer the phone as if everything in the world is normal, to buy groceries as if we will live long enough to eat them, to deal with the life and death issues 24 hours a day, *as if* we will live and not die.

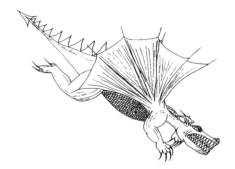

20

No Reconstruction

Feeling Whole
Without It

Since I returned from the hospital, I'd been comforted by the thought that the doctors would create a new breast for the vacancy left there by surgery. Learning to use a silicone prosthesis had posed a number of challenges. Since it was not attached to anything, just inserted inside my bra form, it seemed to develop a playful mind of its own, which posed some interesting problems.

Running was out of the question. Whenever my feet would touch the ground, the prosthesis, which at this point we were all calling my *jelly boob,* would bounce upward, turning slightly with each bounce until the prosthesis would either pop completely out of the bra, or simply land in an odd-looking position. I tried using a cotton covering, pinning it to my bra, but the weight of this free-floating missile simply took over when any motion began.

Weeding in the garden was a challenge. Bending over was impossible, since the prosthesis would slip—ker-plop!—out of the bra form, landing like an oversized beanbag in my shirt, the weight of it making my shirt swing from side to side like an elephant's trunk. I would quickly look around, take off my gardening glove, slip my *boob* back in place, then go on weeding like nothing in the world had happened. My kids became accustomed to this odd scenario, and would just say, "Mo...om!" in an embarrassed fashion. I would just chuckle and go on, wondering what the neighbors thought I was doing to myself. They never asked, and I never offered to explain. (This is one of those "unexpected" challenges tacked onto recoveries, that is never mentioned in the small print.)

Even during normal everyday working hours, the prosthesis would continue to turn in place, presenting the shape of my left breast to the world in many imaginative forms. It was not unusual to answer the door, only to discover that my breast was posing at a 90 degree angle.

Swimming with a prosthesis held its own surprises. The first day back, I took off swimming slowly across the pool, when—POP!—out danced my swimming prosthesis from inside my swim suit! I watched with disbelief as it bobbed jauntily along in front of me. Retrieving this now detachable part of myself, I popped it back into my suit. No men in sight, thank God! I had comical visions of having to call for the male lifeguard to save my floating boob.

Another morning in the pool, I had a completely different experience. Suddenly, I stopped in the middle of a stroke. I caught my breath sharply. It felt like someone had kicked me in the stomach—that deep, sad, scary feeling that comes with a cold sweat when you hear someone you care deeply about is dead.

A deep sadness emanated from the center of my physical being—an oddly familiar mourning sensation. I found myself responding to that physical dimension in words and supportive meanings.

"It's okay," I said. "I understand your sadness. I felt that way, too. You'll be all right. It's okay." For several minutes I spontaneously kept up this supportive discourse, until gradually, the feeling of deep distress passed. I stopped the discourse, and finished my laps. It was extraordinary. It was as though I could feel my physical body reaching out across a chasm of the unknown, the unfamiliar, to my mind and my heart for comfort.

For months I had talked to my body in physical therapy, encouraging it to get well. But this was different. This time I felt my body actually "talking back" to me in a language of feelings and meanings.

I tried to imagine what this might mean to human beings as a whole. Could it be possible that our bodies are made up of interactive layers, able to communicate separately in some meaningful way with us?

I could not deny what had happened, but I did not have any ready explanation for the phenomenon. I realized at that moment that I had mourned the loss of my breast at several levels: spiritually, mentally, emotionally, and now, physically. Not only my arm and the wounded area, but my total physical plane seemed to be processing the loss.

All of life seems so connected, I thought. So connected.

One Sunday morning I awoke to a new thought emerging: *I feel whole!* My body tingled with this new sensation. *I feel complete—even without my breast.* Somehow I felt I no longer needed a reconstructed breast to feel whole again. I stepped back from this new thought, turning it over and over in my mind, until I became quite comfortable with its implications.

No reconstruction means—no more surgery! I told myself. No more surgery means—no more pain to recover from!

Questions I had had since the beginning of the idea of an implant surfaced: Would there be complications? Would an implant age well with me? Perhaps it would be fine at age 44, but what about when I was 82? How much is really known about the safety of such an implant?

I had been informed by a nurse that the implant used was normally filled with a saline solution presently, instead of silicone, which had proven to be a problem in the past when there was a leak. The saline solution was thought to be safer.

How many surgeries would actually be necessary to complete reconstruction? It was my understanding, speaking to others who had had it done, that there was possibly more than one surgery involved. Did I really want to deal with more surgeries, when my inner need to have the breast replaced was no longer there?

For the next few days, I continued to explore the idea of reconstruction. "I think I can handle a permanent prosthesis, without any problem," I relayed to Ellie. "Remember when you mentioned spiritual healing for Jan, even though physically she was lost to cancer?"

"Yes," she responded.

"Well, I thought of your words when this new feeling of whole-ness came. It's like it doesn't matter. I feel good about myself and my body. I'd like to give it a chance to get totally well again. Just a shot at that is an exhilarating feeling."

"You've been through a lot," she said. "You owe it to yourself."

"I could get several prostheses—a furry one for winter, a cotton one for summer…a leafy one for fall…and a flowered one for spring." I chuckled.

"Why not?" Ellie giggled on the other end of the line.

I knew I was all right when I could have fun with the idea. When the news came from our new insurance company that they would not cover a reconstruction since they had not covered the original mastectomy, I decided to take the leap. I understood it was a risk. At some point in the future I might wish I had had it done. I decided to let the future take care of itself. The decision was right for now. I relayed my wishes to Dr. Lennard. Surprised, and appearing somewhat disappointed with my decision, he respectfully accepted it.

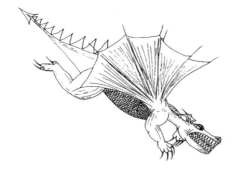

21

Dying and Living

Choosing To Live

Some people die easily, giving in gracefully, while others fight death with every gasp of breath they have. What makes them want life so much?

During my college days, I worked in a nursing home for a year. Some residents faced enormous pain. They were utterly frustrated with how little they were able to accomplish in a day. At some point life was simply no longer worthwhile. Yet, when death offered them release from their misery and pain, it was not unusual to see them resist it with every last bit of energy they had. Curious.

I remember Fred, who was thin as a bone, hated the food, the nurses, his family who never visited him, and at times had to be strapped down to a chair due to his violent outbursts. When he became ill near the end, the inside of his mouth was red and swollen. I remember watching one "experienced" nurse's aide force feeding him orange juice into that sensitive area as he fought her hefty strength.

"Fred, stop it!" she yelled viciously at him, pinning down his arms so that she could more easily continue the torture of pouring the biting juice down his puffy mouth.

New at the job, I stood at the door, horrified. Though Fred clenched his teeth, the aide managed with persistence to completely empty the glass of liquid into his mouth. My mind sped forward to the next feeding, and the next, and the next...

Not long afterwards, Fred left his daily torture in that nursing home. I was with him for part of the night he died. It was my first death. He lay on the bed staring up at the ceiling. Then, for a while, he sat upright—his breathing labored, his color pale gray. For a day-and-a-half, Fred lay struggling against the death that offered him release. I was amazed at his resistance in the face of what he had been through. What did he have to live for?

Only one patient did I see happy to die—a hermit who had lived for years in the mountains around Ellensburg by himself, one of the most contented and intriguing people I ever met. At 94 years old, he had a honey business, caring for a number of bee hives in the nearby hills.

The bane of his life was his stay in the nursing home, made necessary by a broken hip after a fall near his home. The loss of privacy and the inability to make independent decisions was almost more than he could bear. One night his heart acted up, and they thought he was gone, only to have him be revived, and ready and able to tell his tale of life on the other side.

"We are like the flowers," he said fervently the next day. His eyes were deep pools of reflection. "When we die," he announced decisively, "we just die and are no more. We are so pig-headed and full of ourselves that we think we can't die like the animals and plants, but we do." He stroked his long white beard. "It was wonderful, dying. There was no more pain! I'm not afraid to die. I'm ready to go now. I'm getting too old to live in the mountains—I might fall again. The last time I fell I laid there for over half a day before my friend found me.

"But, living in this nursing home is hell! They don't let you do anything for yourself!" He bent his head in my direction, and spoke in a whisper.

"What's the worst is all those preachers who come around trying to convert me, and force me to confess before I die. They're like buzzards. They come every day, never miss a day." His blue-green eyes twinkled like stars.

"I fool 'em. If I hear 'em comin', I just play like I'm sleepin' and pretty soon they go away."

Each day when I finished with my work, I'd sit in his little room and listen to this man of the mountains. I felt very privileged to be the one to hear his song.

For me, death was a tug, a strong magnetic pull inviting me to relinquish my hold on life. The pull was so powerful that at times I found myself staring down a long tunnel. When the pain was intense, the tunnel appeared black and menacing. When the pain resided, the tunnel appeared full of light and comfort—beautiful, hard to say "no" to.

"Mom," Brian said one day, looking down at the back of my hand. "Your hand is starting to look old. Look!" he said with alarm, observing how my skin was beginning to look wrinkled, and my veins were beginning to protrude noticeably. "See mine," he showed me his young hand, skin smooth and flawless.

"I know, Bri. I remember looking at my mother's hands when I was about your age, and seeing the same thing. It's strange to see the same wrinkling in my own hand, and the age spots starting. I wish I could live to see all the wonders you are going to see in your lifetime."

"Bri, I am not going to leave you now. I am *determined* to get well." I said earnestly. "It may take a while, but I'm going to make it!" I looked over to see if my words had alleviated his sense of urgency about my hands looking so old. Head drooping into my lap, he absorbed my words reluctantly.

"We've been through a lot together, haven't we, Bri?" I prodded gently.

"Uh-huh," he whispered, not moving his head.

"Not many moms can say their children saved their lives, can they?" I ruffled his hair.

"No."

"Do you have any idea just how proud of both of you I am? And how much more special life is to me since you saved my life?" I asked, thinking of the night just six months before when I couldn't catch my breath as I was recovering from bronchitis.

I had been sitting in our old lounge chair in the living room, when suddenly my breathing became shallower and shallower, until I found myself gasping for air. Attempting to stay calm, I turned to Monica.

"I'm having—trouble getting—my breath," I said with great difficulty. I reached for the phone and dialed 911. I had the strangest feeling as I pressed the numbers that this was all a dream. Should I really be calling an aid car? What if this wasn't that serious?

"This is not a valid address," the switchboard operator said crisply when I gave her our address. "I have a map in front of me, and it's not on here."

"'York' I gasped, "is the old name—for—35th S.E." I began methodically giving her the directions, hoping she would somehow connect with something I said.

"I'm still not sure, but I'm sending a truck. It's on its way," I heard her say at some point on the other end of the line.

Moni grabbed a flashlight in her hand, running out into the dark night by the road, frantically waving her small arms back and forth, trying to show the firemen where we lived.

Brian grabbed a kitchen chair, scooting it right behind me so that I could sit down at the top of the stairs.

I felt Brian's warm hand in mine as I pressed it tightly. His presence helped calm me as I labored more and more with each breath. "You can do it, Mom," he said over and over, pressing hard on my hand. "You're gonna be all right." I held onto his small hand for dear life. I could see Moni's flashlight beaming back and forth through the front door. Finally the fire truck turned into our driveway, and the welcome team of medics rushed up the stairs.

Moni, Bri and I had worked together like a well-rehearsed team. I was exceedingly proud of their efforts.

"I don't want you to get old," Brian said quietly, as he looked again at my hands. "I wish you could live forever and never die. I'll miss you!" He leaned his young head into the circle of my arms.

"I'm going to live a long, long time, Bri," I said reassuringly. "I'm too ornery to die!

"You'll probably be a daddy, and have a family of your own by that time. And you'll be better prepared for it. But I'll always be with you, because our memories of each other are so strong, and we've shared so many special things together. Even after I die, my spirit will still live, and I will still help you and Moni in any way I can, because I love you...very much. You'll see."

I would like a beautiful blossom for every time I made the decision to live. They would fill my house and overflow into the streets. It was a thousand decisions, sometimes many in one day. It does not surprise me that someone with cancer would eventually give up. What does surprise me is the tenacity of the human spirit to fight something so overwhelming, knowing there are no guarantees in the end. Amazing. I feel privileged to have experienced that aspect of being human.

So, Cancer, here's to life! So there!

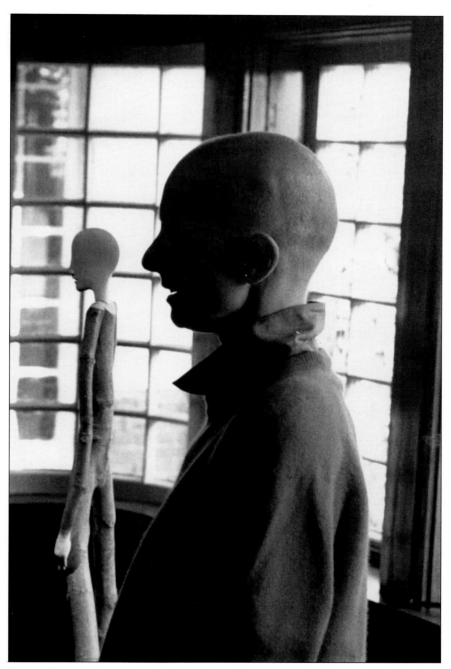

Breast Cancer

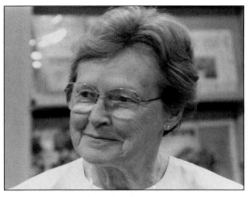

Florence Hannah, retired
Diagnosed 69 years, now 71 years

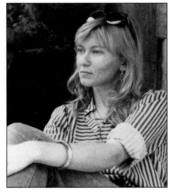

Tara Havemeyer,
  physical therapist
Diagnosed 33 years,
  died 35 years

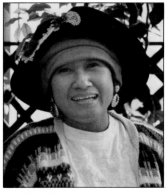

Debbie Collier,
  restaurant owner
Diagnosed 43 years,
  now 44 years

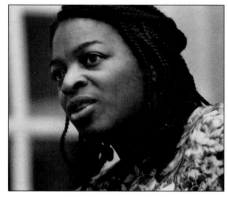

Frenchie Williams, legal assistant
Diagnosed 37 years, now 40 years

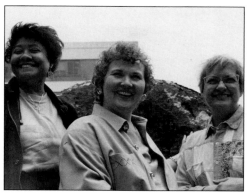

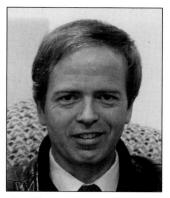

Dr. Thomas Dawson,
family physician

Cora Hill, decorator
Diagnosed 48 years, now 49 years
   Linda Kriede, analyst
   Diagnosed 50 years, now 50 years
      Trudy Bendix, day care provider
      Diagnosed 47 years, now 50 years

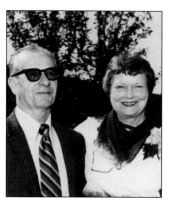

Marie Baker, teacher
  (with husband Bill)
Diagnosed 69 years,
   died 75 years

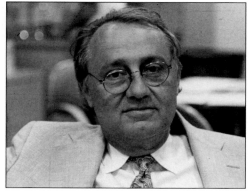

Dr. David Asmussen, D.O., Ob/Gyn.

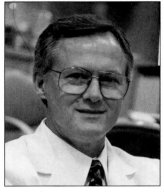

Dr. E. Stan Lennard,
general surgeon

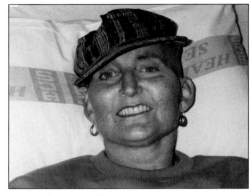

Penny Schick, office manager
Diagnosed 41 years, died 44 years

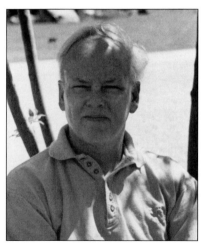

Stephen Meredith,
high school counselor
Diagnosed 46 years,
now 47 years

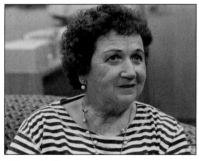

Georgia Fawcett,
nursing assistant
Diagnosed 56 years,
now 66 years

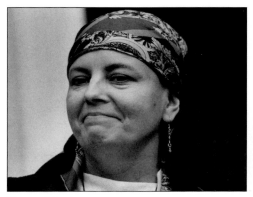

Teresa Martinez
Diagnosed 34 years, now 35 years

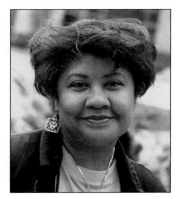

Cora Hill, decorator
Diagnosed 48 years,
    now 49 years

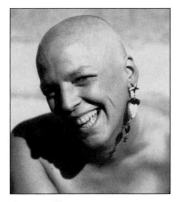

Annette Porter,
    photographer,
    business consultant
Diagnosed 32 years,
    now 35 years

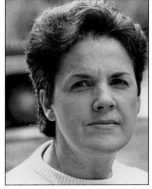

Priscilla McCarty, secretary
Diagnosed 44 years,
    now 50 years

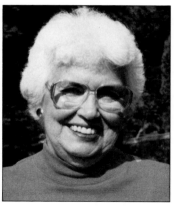

Marie McClintock
Diagnosed 61 years,
died 70 years

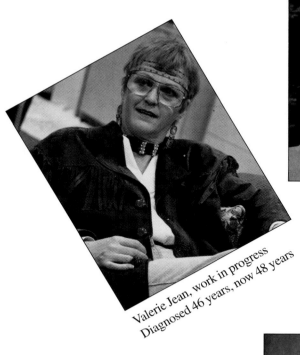

Valerie Jean, work in progress
Diagnosed 46 years, now 48 years

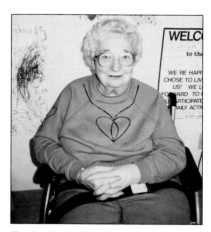

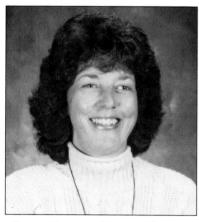

Sharon Harnden, library assistant
Diagnosed 45 years,
now 51 years

Evelyn Frazell, retired teacher
Diagnosed 75 years,
now 77 years

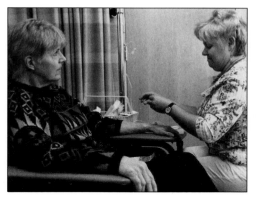

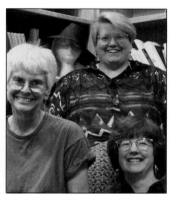

Sharon McKee, business owner
Diagnosed 52 years, now 54 years

Elaine Lachlan,
 social oncologist
Sandra Johnson,
 supervisor,
 cancer support services
Judy Jones,
 cancer education
 specialist

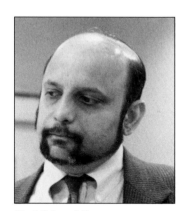

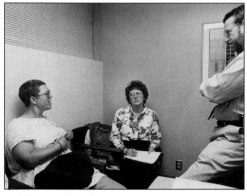

Dr. Mukund Sargur,
 oncologist, hematologist,
 internist

Kathryn Gunther
Diagnosed 42 years, now 44 years
Clo Wilson-Hashiguchi
Diagnosed 44 years, now 50 years
Dr. Thomas Johnson,
 radiation oncologist

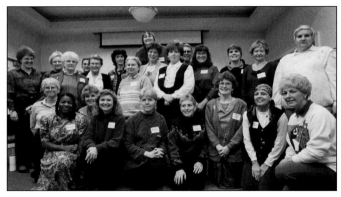

"Bosom Buddies" breast cancer support group
Kirkland, Washington

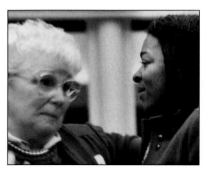

Evelyn Driscoll
Diagnosed 66 years,
    now 70 years
Frenchie Williams
Diagnosed 37 years,
    now 40 years

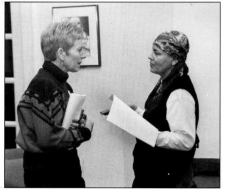

Linda Fankhauser
Diagnosed 45 years, now 50 years
    Teresa Martinez
        Diagnosed 34 years, now 35 years

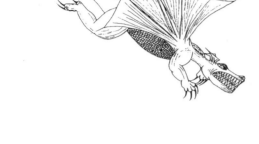

Epilogue

January 1995. It is six years this last November since I had breast cancer. I'm cancer-free so far. It is such a precious thing, well-being. Now I am aware of making choices every day that support health in all aspects of my life.

I no longer hurry so. I know I often need to rest, rejuvenate, and just be still. So I've cut my obligations in half, and I've doubled the time I allow to do the things I choose to do. I am more selective about what I say yes to, and before I commit myself I usually take time to "percolate" on it first, away from the immediate situation, to reflect on how it fits into the rest of my life.

I've started a garden. Flowers bloom everywhere, and every day I walk out to sample the gifts from the fruit trees, berry bushes of all sorts, and my vegetable garden, where there is corn, lettuce, zucchini, and even a pumpkin patch in the fall.

Glenn and I are parting ways. A most difficult, healthy decision. In many ways, he and I are doing better than we ever have, on behalf of ourselves and our children. Strange that such a decision would bring health into our lives, but it has. The difficulties of being together did not go away with breast cancer, though there was a momentary reprieve during my illness.

Monica and Brian are now 16 and 15 years old, vibrant and creative. They show courage in taking risks, as they explore and grow daily as human beings. The kids and I have gone through counseling to process what has happened, so we can go on with our lives. In a very good way, it has helped us process what the experience of my breast cancer meant to each of us. Counseling has helped us let go of what has happened, so that we can be open to all life has to offer us from this point on.

Life is an extraordinary journey. I appreciate each day I'm alive. Let's celebrate!

Stealing the Dragon's Fire
Clo Wilson-Hashiguchi

Part II
Interviews

Marie and Bill Baker
Stephen Meredith
Dr. Mukund Sargur

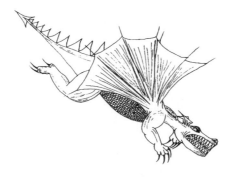

Marie Baker with Husband, Bill

Taped Interview April 27, 1990

The morning I drove south to Enumclaw was clear and sunny. I was taken with the friendly two-lane country road weaving in and out through the expansive miles of farmland, a pleasant contrast to busy urban areas nearby.

I had heard about Marie Baker from her daughter Marleen, who mentioned that her mother was handling her mastectomy well. I asked to meet her, with the possibility of interviewing her for this book. Soon I arrived at Marie and Bill's front door, which opened to one of the most delightful days I have ever spent.

Marie was one of those gentlewomen whose strong, dependable character flavored all she said and did, without taking from her generous spirit.

Though having a mastectomy is a private affair, Marie shared her thoughts openly and generously. An articulate woman, she evoked respect in the way she personally defined this delicate subject.

Marie: When you're first told you have cancer, you go into shock. You don't hear everything the doctors are saying. I'd been checked by our family doctor. All of a sudden there was a little spot on my breast, and within a week it was an ugly red. The tumor was right there on the outside. I had a terrible ache in my arms and I could hardly turn my head.

That was during the same week I had bone scans done. The lump changed, my breast changed, and I knew what I had. But what I didn't expect was for the doctor to say I had bone cancer, too.

Bill: He called Monday and told us he wanted to see us the next day. We went to his office, and that's when he told us the results of the bone scan. She was operated on the next day—Wednesday.

M: It was very fast. I didn't have to think about it. When the doctor told me I had bone cancer—that was the death sentence in my mind. He also told me that I still needed the mastectomy—if I still wanted it. I told him I don't want this breast. It's not good. If people like me for that, they're going to have to get acquainted with somebody else. We're more than just parts of our body.

Our daughter Joanne works at the same clinic, and I went to see her. I opened my mouth to tell the news, but no words came out! That never happened to me before! We just wrapped our arms around each other and cried. She took me in a private room and we cried and cried and cried. I even forgot about Bill. Maybe he was in shock, too. About 15 minutes later, I told Joanne that we'd cried enough. But we got it out of our system. I went back to my doctor's office, and I told him that I just couldn't talk! He said that it was shock and was natural.

Clo: The doctor chose to take care of the mastectomy first?

M: Yes. He said that we will know what to do later. I just accepted that at the time, because I didn't know what would have to be done. I knew I had to get rid of the cancerous breast.

C: Did they say anything about the lymph nodes at that time?

M: Oh, they took them out. Before the operation he told me that they still would send the tissue to the lab, and if they found that it was what they thought it was—cancer—I'd wake up without a breast. I understood that.

C: He didn't do any biopsy before you went in?

M: No, he just put me in that operating room right there and then. They could tell by the looks of it—the nipple was changing. There was good proof. It happened so fast. Some cancers do that.

After the operation when a nurse was giving me a shot, in came the sweetest little cancer lady to tell me about exercising and other things. She had a little kit—a small rubber ball, a little pillow, and some string with two tongue depressors attached.

The doctor let me exercise a little bit in the hospital. When I got home I put a mark with Bon Ami on the sliding door to the bathtub, and every day I would move my arm up, and when the pain started, I'd stop. That way I could see the improvement. It was a little encouragement. When I was healed, I asked my doctor if I could I go swimming. He let me go swimming—three weeks after surgery!

I'm more of a dog-paddler, but I've made up my own little strokes. It brought my arm out. I had been swimming with the same ladies for almost five years, and one day one woman came up to me in the dressing room and told me she didn't think I knew how to fix my swimsuit.

She showed me how to put a pocket for the prosthesis in my swimsuit. And then she said to go ahead and take a shower and not to hide. She helped me a lot to get over my shyness. Swimming got me back to reality much faster. So many people were encouraging me.

C: How has it been for you, Bill?

B: It hurts. We'll do what we have to do.

M: I have a lot of good days. And I enjoy them. The two days right after chemo aren't too good. I know that, and I plan dinners for that. Bill will eat his meal, but I just go in the bedroom and sleep it off.

C: Are you just about finished with your chemo?

M: I don't know. They won't tell me. It's holding. The doctor doesn't want to rock the boat. He said I'm doing so well. I haven't had a bone scan now for a while.

C: How is a bone scan done?

M: Well, it's a very funny machine. It's huge. And, you're hoping that bolt above you holds.

C: It's right over the top of you?

M: You bet it is. You're lying on this cold slab. [Chuckle] You think may be you're already gone beyond! The machine has a little teeny set on which you can see flickering—flick, flick, flick. It looks like a TV set. The technicians set it and run out of the room. You count about 20 seconds, and you hear a click, and you know they've taken a picture.

C: So, it's just like having an X-ray?

M: It's different. When I have a bone scan at 10 in the morning, I have to go in at about 7:30 or 8, and they shoot me with radioisotopes. Then I have to drink a tall glass of pink stuff, and they send me home. I have to drink eight glasses of anything I want so that the chemicals get into the bones.

B: The cancer shows up black on the X-ray.

C: Where did they find your bone cancer?

B: In the ribs.

M: There was one that showed up right here [pointing to her clavicle], here, here, here [pointing to various spots on her upper body].

B: She has some on the top, various spots on her ribs, her spine. Her major bones are relatively free.

M: My legs seem to be pretty clear, but it's in the hip bones. It's in my whole system, but it's holding. Nothing new has shown up since I've been on chemo.

C: Marleen suggested that there might have been a place where you were working that had something in the structure—asbestos, that might have contributed to your getting cancer?

M: Well, it could have been asbestos in the school. I don't know.

B: It could have happened during the year-and-a-half when I was overseas, from '44 to '46, when she lived in Ellensburg. This is a supposition—the radioactive stuff in the air from the Tri-Cities. That's still a question.

M: We had a day in Ellensburg when anything on the clothesline that was nylon disappeared!

B: It just disintegrated.

C: Disintegrated?

M: Yes, they never could answer the questions we all had.

B: It's still being questioned.

M: I always thought it was some kind of cloud that must have gone over us. It was about 1945.

B: They don't want the responsibility.

C: Did it happen any more than once?

M: No, I just remember that one time. Mother and I had hardly anything on the clothesline. Annie M. called, and said, "Don't hang anything out! It'll disappear!" All the nylons were GONE!

C: Were there any other teachers who worked with you who got cancer?

M: There are a lot of teachers who have had cancer. We're just amazed by it.

C: Do some have cancer who taught in the same place you taught?

M: Yes: Beata. She taught second grade. And, Margaret just passed away. She taught first grade. And, some of our high school teachers have had cancer.

B: The art teacher in high school.

M: And then, Mrs. Alsgaard.

B: There are several others.

M: I have a theory about cancer. I feel we all have cancer cells in our bodies. If something goes wrong, the body can't control it, then the cancer gets control. But somehow it's there, and it comes out in different forms in different people. What causes it? I don't think they know. Stress may have something to do with it, but I never was too stressed.

C: You don't feel like your cancer was caused by stress?

M: I don't think so. We've handled our stress pretty well. Bill was in the war [World War II] for two years and I was alone with Marleen. That was a stressful time. But we all have stress we have to handle.

C: Do you think it might have been some kind of environmental cause that might have triggered?

M: I don't think so. I really don't. I just think it was something my own body couldn't handle. I don't know.

C: How old were you when you had your mastectomy?

M: It was three years ago. I was 69.

C: Is there a history of cancer in your family?

M: I couldn't find any. Women didn't write things down in my mother's generation. And if they did know, they wouldn't tell anybody. I wrote to one of my aunts, and all she said was: "Hmph! Hmph! Hmph!" I thought, okay, I'm through with you!

I always suspected that Aunt Alta might have had it. They said that she had appendicitis. But later on, when I got older and knew more, I discovered she had a hysterectomy. They didn't talk about those things. My father had cancer of the duodenum. But first he had cancer of the nose.

He had a little sore in his nose, and they gave him radiation. He was 75 when that cleared up. He was just perkin' right along until he was over 92. He just thought he had a little stomach problem that milk of magnesia would cure. But that wasn't it. He was diagnosed June 7. He chose not to have an operation. He passed away three weeks later. He had a long, healthy life. The end was quick.

C: You mentioned Joanne, and I've met Marleen. How many children do you have?

M: We have three girls. Marleen's the oldest, then Joanne, and then Sandy. They're all in Washington. We have five grandchildren: two granddaughters and three grandsons. I have a good, supportive family and friends.

When I was first diagnosed with cancer, they started me out on two different pills that worked well—Nolvadex and Megace. But then, I could tell something was wrong and I went to the doctor. He suggested a change and put me on chemo or radiation, or both. I went through a CAT Scan, a bone scan, and a sound scan—all those machines! Something new was added. He told me that my veins would collapse with time and recommended I get a "Port-a-Cath." [She opened her blouse, pointing to a small apparatus below the skin.] They poke right through there [pointing to an opening] and attach it to a vein, and administer my chemo that way.

C: Did you have to go through a surgical procedure to get it inserted?

M: Yes. I had a local anesthetic. But, I told the doctor I didn't want to watch it. He told me he would put sheets in front of me, and would talk to me the whole time. That was all right.

C: How long have you had the Port-a-Cath?

M: It's been in a year. I have two very good chemo nurses who usually give me my chemo. They use me as a "guinea pig" sometimes, because they've been training other hospital nurses to give chemo. They come over, because I have a Port-a-Cath, and teach them how to do it. They've had me show people who are going to get a "port," and tell them before an operation to relax, so they're not frightened. I even had to show it to a man, once.

C: How about your lymph nodes? Did they find some involvement of cancer?

M: Yes. They took out a whole lot. [NOTE: *They took all the lymph nodes on the left side. All were involved.*—Marleen]

C: Did the doctors determine that the bone cancer was metastasized breast cancer?

M: Yes, it came from the breast and went to the bones.

C: Have you had radiation treatment?

M: No. I developed quite a pain in my right hip, just when this other medicine [the pills] had stopped working. The doctor said that we may have to do radiation. I went through the X-ray routine again when he said we'd do the chemo. When I went home that night I didn't have any pain in my hip. The chemo did it. I had no aches and no pains.

C: When you go in for a chemo treatment, what are your thoughts?

M: Because it has helped the cancer, I just figure it's something I have to do. I'm afraid if I don't have it, I might develop something else. I can take two days of not feeling well because it's helping me, I think. Also, I try to eat right.·

C: Have you changed your diet?

M: No, we've always eaten just "good old" food—lots of vegetables.

C: Have you taken any extra vitamins?

M: No, I don't take anything. And, I can't have any aspirin-based products with my chemo. I can't have any liver, but I never did eat it anyway. And I've never smoked.

C: What do you think you've learned from having cancer?

M: Well, your values change. Small things become big—your family for one thing. There may be some unfinished business, and all of a sudden you want to finish things. I have these Grandmother books which I want to complete for each grandchild. Little things like getting the picture books up to date for the girls. Things that I used to think were important have gotten into perspective. They're not that important.

C: Why do you think that is?

M: Well, you know, you've got to face the door of death for one thing. Of course, it's there all the time for everybody, but people aren't aware of it. We're all going to die.

C: What do you think is the toughest part of having cancer?

M: I think the fatigue has been the hardest. I don't have that as much now, but just walking across the room—I could hardly walk across the room and walk back again!

C: Was that before the surgery or after?

M: No, that was after. Actually it was really after the chemo.

C: And now?

M: After the chemo I'm not as tired now. I think they found a good formula for me. My hair was thinning, but it never all came out. And, now it's growing and getting thick again. In fact, I have to have a haircut about every month now. I bought two wigs immediately. They're my insurance policy. It would have been the hardest trauma, to be a "baldy." Also, I've stayed away from people who've had sadness.

C: Would you explain what you mean?

M: I got myself in a frame of mind to be happy, and that feels good. Why would I do anything to be unhappy?

C: Are you saying that it added to your sadness if other people were unhappy?

M: Well yes, if they started crying it bothered me—like when a baby cries. I couldn't help them and they weren't helping me. This was not the case with my family, but with the people from the support groups.

C: Do you mean cancer support groups?

M: Yes. That's why I wouldn't go to meetings. The Cancer Society gave me books to read, and Marleen and I discuss some of the books. Sandy and all the girls—including my niece, who is very close to me— kept up.

C: Were you all reading these books at the same time?

M: Yes. Then they wrote letters and called me on the telephone. I had a lot of support. But my older brother needed some help and I knew I was going to have to do something. He didn't come to see me. He wasn't calling. I thought he was in shock. He'd lost two wives to cancer. His sister had cancer. That was hard. I finally called him and I told him, "Get off your duff and come on over! I want to see you."

He wanted to know if I was feeling all right and if he could come. I told him he'd better come. The moment he saw me, he was all right. But he was moping around and worrying. Later, I read in one of those books, "Sometimes you have to help your relatives." I had already done it! I could've written a book, I guess. I had to help him over the hump.

There's a lot of misinformation about cancer in our heads. Where we got it, we don't know, but it's there, and we have to filter that out.

Then, I realized that we were paying a doctor, and he was going to have to answer my questions. Nobody else was. He's been educated. If he doesn't know, he'll refer me to somebody who does. I have complete faith in my doctor. He's a good doctor.

C: Are there parts of what you've gone through with cancer that you have had to do by yourself—without family or friends?

M: Well, you do feel alone. You feel like you're in a box. You're fighting to get the lid open. Faith and prayers help an awful lot. I just feel that when the Lord dishes it out, he's not going to give you any more than you can handle. And I think you have to take care of yourself. When you're tired, then you'd better say no. If you don't want people around, then you'd better say no. If I'm on the telephone with a long-winded person, and my arm gets tired, I say, "I can't talk any more. My arm is tired."

I've always been independent, but I think I'm a little more so now—thinking of me, thinking of myself. When I get tired, I just excuse myself and lie down. I don't care if we have a whole house full of company. I'm tired and they've got to accept it. I'm not faking it. When I'm rested, I'm zipping around. It's a different tiredness.

C: How would you describe it?

M: It hits you out of the blue. You never know when. That's why you don't plan too far ahead, like a long shopping trip, or going out. You just don't plan to get too far away from home. I don't, because it might hit, and then there's nothing I can do. I just have to sleep.

C: You were talking about pain in your arm. Have you had problems with pain when your arm gets cold?

M: No, and I think that's because I go swimming, and I do exercises. The doctors have asked me if I've had numbness, cold, or swelling. Well, I know that I can never have anything taken out of this arm.

C: You mean, in terms of IV's?

M: Yes. Once, one little guy did. I was having a CAT Scan. The young man took out the IV for his convenience, because he had all these instruments to handle. I told him that he couldn't take it out of this arm. Well, he did anyway and I ended up with phlebitis. I also have to be careful about being in the sun with chemo. I don't dare get sunburn. I keep out of the sun and use a sunscreen.

C: What is supposed to happen?

M: It makes you sick. Your skin burns too deep and you don't feel it. Another thing to avoid are products containing alcohol. I threw away Listerine, and other stuff. I checked all my cosmetics. I can't have any alcohol on my face or skin. I use soda for mouth wash, or just water. I read my literature real well. I had kids to get well for. I want to see these grandkids growing up. I had a lot of motivation.

C: The people in our lives don't have any idea how important they are in motivating us to get well, do they?

M: No. I want you to see something. [She leads me into an adjacent room, pointing to a striking painting of a landscape.] I sat down and painted that picture the day before my operation.

C: You did!

M: It helped. It passed the time, and I wasn't worrying about the operation.

C: It's beautiful, Marie. That's interesting, because my writing helps me keep my balance. Have you felt like your music has helped you, too?

M: Oh, yes. I sang in the community chorus. We did beautiful programs. I was still in the chorus when I was on the pill chemo, but as soon as I was on the shot chemo, I had to get out. Then I had to quit teaching. But I went back and subbed— those little kids just loved me. They didn't know there was anything wrong with me. I did tell them that my arm had been operated on, which was true. My little reading group was so nice. When I got up, they put my chair and my book away.

C: It sounds like they wanted to take good care of you.

M: I don't think some things are as important anymore. Life passes by. You've got to reach for the goodies. Another thing to do is to read the good books the Cancer Society has available, and not to be afraid to call the Cancer Society for help. If a person has a financial problem, they provides free wigs, free prostheses, and a lot of things.

The last time I went for treatment, there was a long table set up with a whole bunch of wigs and a sign that said: "Free Wig. Take the one you like." People who didn't need a wig anymore had turned them in.

C: A prosthesis is quite expensive ($190 to $300 each). In terms of cost, what about the built-in Sears bras you mentioned?

M: Bill, do you remember how much those Sears bras were?

B: Two of them run around $142 and you can get them from Sears Shop At Home service.

C: I didn't know a built-in bra was even available.

[Note: Available through Sears Shop At Home service. See Bibliography.]

M: I had a squeaky prosthesis!

C: A squeaky one?

M: Yes. This was really funny. I was squeaking!

C: When would it squeak?

M: At any moment! Everyone in the family thought it was ha-ha funny. But, it wasn't funny to me. People were looking around to see where the squeaking came from. It was time to buy a couple new bras and we went to Nordstrom. I just casually told the salesperson that my prosthesis squeaks.

The young girl said, "Well, that's not right. It's the fluid—it's just getting "fluidy."

She asked me if had worn the prosthesis on an airplane. I told her that when I have to fly, I just use the ones I've made that are stuffed with cotton.

B: Some women with silicone implants have had trouble on a plane. The implants would expand with the altitude.

C: That sounds painful!

M: Yes! It is also embarrassing. I didn't want that to happen to me. The clerk said the prosthesis was defective. She gave me a brand new one—no questions asked.

C: Have you ever considered reconstruction?

M: No, I'm too old for that. I only wanted to go through this ordeal once.

C: If you could share some thoughts with someone who had just been informed that she has cancer, what would you say to her?

M: I'd tell her not to be afraid, for one thing and to put herself into the hands of a doctor she feels safe with. Then she should be completely relaxed and do everything she's told to do. Listen to the professional people. And, when she gets emotional, if she's alone, she can call someone she is close to and talk about her feelings.

C: Reach out?

M: Reach out; try not to be inward. You get morbid when you do that. Pretty soon the whole world gets you down. You start asking yourself why is this happening to you, and you get too engrossed in your own feelings. When you go for chemo you see other people worse off than you are. You're pretty darn glad you're where you are. Some people are in pretty bad shape. And when you don't see them any-more—you know why. But, there's also a cheerfulness—after a while you can pin-point cancer patients. They have such a good outlook. That comes with the cancer.

C: Why do you say that comes with the cancer?

M: Because the only thing you can control is your own personal-ity. You can't control your physical being, but you can control your emotional being. It helps to listen to other people, get involved and help them. By helping them, you help yourself as well. It happened to me at chemo. There was a man who seemed very upset. He had his little chart and other things. I asked him what was bothering him about these papers. He said, that there were too many things to handle. It was too much for him.

I told him not to worry, he wouldn't have to do all those 20 things at once, and I asked him if he had chemo before? He said it was his first time! I said, "Don't be surprised if you get sick. Don't fight it, just be sick. Get it over with. And then, when you get well, you're going to feel all right." It seemed to help him.

I kept a daily log of reactions and my feelings, and what had hap-pened with the different chemos. I could then pinpoint when I was get-ting too much and when I wasn't getting enough. I'd tell the doctor and he would adjust the chemo so I wouldn't get so sick. It helped a lot.

C: What an excellent idea!

M: People who have cancer shouldn't feel that it hasn't happened to anybody else. It's happened to me. It's happened to a lot of people. Some people who have cancer feel they have to get out of the main-stream. I think you have to get *in* some form of a mainstream.

C: Would you describe more what you mean?

M: Well, I wouldn't give up my substitute teaching. That was my mainstream. I knew when I was able to go. By subbing I could be very selective. I taught for 30 years, plus 10 years of subbing. That's 40 years. I'd take the good classes, and the teachers who planned the best lessons. It was fun. I'd go, and I'd have a good day. It keeps you active—you have to stay active.

C: What would you say about someone who might be too active?

M: I don't think you should overdo. Physically, your body isn't as healthy, and you're not as strong. I think I'm quite lazy! I've learned shortcuts. I saw a book the other day, and it said "Make a dinner in 15 minutes." That's the kind of dinner I like! I think you get selfish about yourself. It's your health, and you want to squeeze every inch out of it when you're feeling good. If you don't feel good, don't feel guilty about it. It might be a warning—maybe you are overdoing. Maybe you need to kick your shoes off and take a nap, rest. But I don't compare myself with other people too much. I'm my own person.

C: Do you think that is significant in terms of your recovery?

M: I think so. It doesn't matter to me if so-and-so thinks my hair is the right color. When the kids visited and we celebrated a birthday, there were 10 people here. I have beautiful dishes, but I decided to use paper plates. We put the paper plates in little baskets and used some other wicker things. It looked like a picnic. The boys were as happy as clams. The only things we used that wasn't paper were the napkins—and the washing machine takes care of them. Everybody was happy, because there weren't a lot of dishes to do. You've just got to keep things easy.

NOTE: *On January 28, 1993, Marie Baker died in the hospital, her body full of cancer, still making her own choices of how to fight it to the end. Two days before she died she elected to have surgery to remove tumors from blocking her kidneys. One of her last wishes was to have her body cremated, so she could finally kill forever every cancer cell in her body. She was a life warrior in the truest sense. We all honor her memory, and what she taught us about living.*

Stephen Meredith

High School Counselor
Taped Interview June 29, 1994

*I found Stephen Meredith to be a remarkable human being—
sensitive, articulate, caring, with a delightful sense of humor—a man
of heart. I honor that Stephen has been willing to step forward to address
the male experience of breast cancer so openly, fully aware that this disease is usually identified as a "woman's disease." His courage to speak
out may create a platform for other men to address more openly the
terror of this disease, reaching out to each other with hope.*

Stephen: I'm trying to understand how I am taking advantage of
who I was before and how I'm handicapped by who I was then. I think
we are a mixture of our strengths and our weaknesses. For instance, I
played basketball in college, and I've always been very competitive.

Clo: How does your competitiveness come into play in terms of
your cancer?

S: Rather than just surviving, I want to beat it—I want to win.
People say I have a good attitude, but I really have no choice. I know I
went into this big-dip decline at the beginning. Everybody has a diagnosis for you, everybody has a solution. I'm basically conservative; I
trust the medical community. In the first few months I was worried
about my life, but in some ways I was also worried about choosing the
right path—the right follow-up treatment. Would it be totally holistic,
would I wear pukka shells? I was wondering what my medical and therapeutic solution would be.

The "dip" manifested itself in the way I was thinking; I planned
for my immediate future: my job, my work with high school kids. I
took several days off for the surgery and five days for recovering. In
addition to that, I was going to pull back and rest. I had a summer holi-
day coming up, but by about the 15th of August, I realized things would
really start heating up again. September and October are my busiest
months of the year in terms of activities, what with homecoming and my

counseling work. I'd be right in the middle of that and I thought, "Screw that." I'm not going to do it. I'm not going to go to school in September because I'd be at the end of my chemotherapy. People told me that when you start chemotherapy, you are really feeling bad by the sixth month. "Whacked out" was how one friend who had chemotherapy after breast cancer surgery described it." I kept remembering that phrase, "Whacked out." But I haven't been "whacked out."

During that "dip," I made plans to miss time at school. I was cocooning, building this little world around me—to protect myself. One thing that was going to protect me was staying away from work. Somehow, I had connected the stress in my work life and the turmoil that goes with teaching to my illness. I was going to cut that out and rest. It would be a time for me to reorder things in my life. Following the diagnosis, I was terribly depressed. But I was probably in shock then. Just the physiological effects do that. People get into a car accident—"Boom." Things close down around them. They go into shock, their blood pressure and their heart rate go way down, which seriously jeopardizes their health. I know that in the same way everything started to close down on me.

C: Do you think understanding what was going on with you helped you recover from that period?

S: I'm not sure. In retrospect I think what happened is that I got through that point. At first I was waiting for the time when I wasn't going to go to work any more, everything was going to be in order, and I would hand it over to somebody else. But I was involved in so many interesting things. I was on several committees and I was running; I was needed. Then in September, there was no question about going to school. It wasn't that I had to—I wanted to.

I was reading Bernie Siegel, and he said that hard work doesn't make you tired. Things you don't like make you tired. Things that are difficult and stressful for you make you tired. The work you enjoy doesn't tire you out. When I read that, I thought, "I'm not tired of what I'm doing, I don't need to get away from it."

Everything was so emotional at the beginning, but now it's better. I just had a nice talk with a fellow who lives in a community just south of here. He said that I'm an example of how to approach a serious illness and a gentle reminder to appreciate life. Others have said to me, "Boy, look at the way you're running your life. You're exercising a lot. You're going on with your life, and you're not letting the treatment for the illness be worse than the illness. You're not letting the spectre of perhaps dying dominate your actions." I watched one of my friends change his life a little bit. He now spends more time with his kids, more time exercising and taking care of himself. It was nothing I said to him.

C: Do you see yourself as an agent of change because of the breast cancer?

S: Not intentionally. During that two-month period when I was closing all the doors and deciding I wasn't going to work, I was probably pretty down. That was natural. I didn't realize it until this woman pointed it out: "Boy you went through that big dip where you closed all the doors." I didn't start boxing stuff up, but the metaphor was there.

C: It sounds like your life was so interesting with so many things going on, that it kept propelling you, bringing you back to living.

S: I think that's really accurate. The fact that I'm able to work around those neat kids and be part of that unbridled enthusiasm has been really fortunate. Had I been a computer analyst or an accountant, maybe I wouldn't have had all that external stimulation.

I told a small group of kids who really needed to know to co-opt a little bit in my grief. I told them because I thought I wouldn't be there in September. Some kids were really sad and some were upset. A lot of 17-, 18-year-old kids have not dealt with the specter of death. For a lot of people, just the cancer diagnosis is a death sentence. The first contact with someone who is ill enough to die is really hard for the kids. But they didn't all react the same way. Some became really motherly: "Get out of here! It's 4:30, what are you doing here? You should be going home, you should be resting!" Some kids didn't say anything, which was okay. The best part of it was, "I know you're sick, but we've got an assembly on Friday. We've got stuff to do." They didn't say out loud, "I know you're sick." Their enthusiasm for life didn't stop because mine was derailed a bit.

It was a little like kids coming home to a mother who is sick and say, "We know you're sick, but we've got to have dinner and you've got to run us to the ball field," and, "Well, you know...life's got to go on."

C: Do you think that's a different experience for a dad than for a mom?

S: That's interesting. I have a bunch of responsibilities around the house—from doing dishes to taking the kids places. My wife and I both work. She does her share as far as income and working goes. I share child care stuff. I'm not just the breadwinner, my wife won't allow that. I've got jobs and she's got jobs. She doesn't stay home all day. We do quite a bit of sharing. I'm not sure how this would affect me differently if I were a woman. I've thought about the prospect of not being here. I'm much more aware now of how much teaching I do with my kids and how much value-structuring I'm trying to impart on them.

C: Does breast cancer alter how you relate to your family?

S: I don't think so. I'm seeing my role with a little more clarity. In some sort of gallows' way, I'm imagining not being here to fulfill that role.

Last night we were having dinner on the patio. My older daughter was trying to cut flank steak with a fork. I showed her how to hold the knife, how to cut, switch hands and where to place the knife. I would have done that any time, but in some way I backed up and began to reflect: "You know, this is why I'm here. This is what's really important." I appreciated it more because of what's happened to me. In some subtle ways, I'm passing on that awareness to my friend who says, "My life is going to be a little bit different from knowing you." Not that I've told him, "You ought to spend a little more time with your daughters, teaching them how to cut meat!" He sees me and he extrapolates, "Boy that person could be dying. He must really value some things in his life now more intensely than ever before. I should do the same." He says I'm now a teacher in a way that I never was before. Sometimes I'll say, "This is what I've learned from this. You need to prioritize things." Sometimes I say things I've been thinking about but never verbalized before, and I say them with a new awareness. I'm almost in a new culture.

C: Is this new awareness the result of facing your mortality?

S: I think that's it. I told my friend that he and I really are no different. Each of us has a time line; I've just have a better glimpse of mine. All of a sudden, I'm aware that the road that I'm on has an end. I think before something like this happens, we all see ourselves as somehow infinitely ageless.

C: Do you think that alters the quality of your life?

S: I definitely think it has. I have been able to step back and realize the impact. I don't think people get a chance often enough to tell others that they care about them, and that they have done some things that were right. If anything, a lot of people have had an opportunity to tell me what they think about me. That's been really nice!

C: Stephen, how old are you?

S: I'm 47.

C: How about your children? How did you handle that part of dealing with cancer that includes your kids?

S: I've talked to them. They know I'm sick, but they also see how well I am. I don't think it's up to me to make it more of an urgent thing, more compelling, more serious or more gripping than it needs to be. It's likely that the cancer is gone from my system, and chemotherapy is going to chase away any bad bugs that are running around, and I'm going to go on. I want them to know that this brush with life—or death—has had a real effect on me. My kids are only eleven and eight and have a limited capacity for understanding that, and I don't see any advantage to making them more aware of the fact that I could die.

C: Do they know you have cancer?

S: Yes. At the time when I was in the hospital sleeping off one of my surgeries, Linda told the girls: "Your dad is really sick, he has cancer. That's why he's upstairs sleeping. They had to do surgery on him and he's going to be a while recovering. He will have some bad scars, but he's going to be okay."

Bridget, my eight-year-old, responded, "Is he going to die?" I mean, that was it—it was either yes or no.

Linda said, "No, he's not going to die; he's going to make it." Part of it was hoping, and part of it was based on the medical diagnosis. That was it, the girls didn't want to talk about it anymore. They wanted to go on with their lives. And I want to let them.

C: So your journey is different from that of your kids?

S: I think so. Obviously it's happening to me and I'm constantly aware of it. I'm more threatened by it personally. One of the things I feel guilty about is that I'm not doing more, I'm not paying more attention to it, maybe like you. You've committed your life to it for the last five years. You've immersed yourself in all of the information you could get and have reached out to so many people and now you're writing a book.

C: Actually that's not exactly true. I started a journal for myself, and this book came out of that. It evolved for other people. It's true that I'm immersed in it, but it's also true that I won't let this book become my life. That's why the book is still growing, why it's not done yet. I won't kill myself to write it. As a result, I have come in contact with a lot more people like you, there has been time for collaboration, and a fabric exists that wouldn't have been there if I hadn't.

S: I went to a natural health conference. I don't know what I expected, but I expected a whole lot more. There were a lot of holistic medicines and herbs, and people who wanted to sell you stuff, rather than teaching you how to go on. I did meet one man and bought his book. I haven't read it yet. I have been too busy living and enjoying myself. I guess I feel a bit guilty that I haven't been more attentive to the other options. Creative visualization. I was doing that in the shower. Things were closed off, and God, I've wasted a lot of water. I don't know what my thing is. I don't want chemotherapy to be my thing. I hope that maybe it's my attitude and I'm doing things already that are really good.

C: It sounds to me like the kids are your thing, and your life is your thing, and your family is your thing, and your friends are your thing. It is such an individual journey. I have observed the people with whom I have talked and those who do best are doing exactly what you are doing, they are choosing their own unique way through it.

S: Bernie Siegel says, "Find your own true path." He says to look back six to eighteen months before you were diagnosed with cancer and see how your life is different. I see some definite changes. I'm a lot different now than I was back then. But I'm not taking herbs, I'm not meditating, I'm not doing a lot of these other options I read about. I know I'll only pass this way once—from early diagnosis to five years out. I'll only be in this slot once. I want to do everything I can, but I can't seem to make myself. I'm too busy enjoying myself and living. I remember a good friend of mine who was in that slot. He tried a lot of things. I'm not sure how intensely he tried them. He eventually died. It was stomach cancer. It was awful.

I'm stepping back and realizing that, at this period, there is a lot of "lobster" in my life. So for me, awareness has been the most profound change. I'm just more aware. Each time I write in my journal, I go back to my calendar and I look at everything that brought me joy and happiness, and I write it down. Just list them: going out to a baseball game, going to Hood Canal, going out with one of my friends and drinking beer. Before, it just happened. All this happiness has always been there before. All of a sudden, I'm aware that happiness is all around me. The paradigm shift is not more happiness for me, but understanding it, and appreciating it.

Is there a chemical difference between a person who goes to a baseball game with friends and whoops it up and the person who goes to a baseball game with friends and whoops it up and reflects on how enjoyable it was?

C: Is there any family history of cancer?

S: None. My father's sister died of lung cancer. She died with eight cigarettes in her mouth, I think. My dad smoked for 50 years, and so did my mom. They quit ten or fifteen years ago. They're both 82 and are still plugging along.

C: Any risk factors?

S: We had barbecued steak last night, and we probably have red meat once a month, maybe three times a month—but not very often. We eat a lot of chicken, and Linda has her garden. I broke my neck in a car accident and I have a bad back. I wonder about the effect of nerve damage. I played a lot of basketball and got hit on top of my head a lot; I'm sure I hurt myself. Then I started running—all that pounding on the pavement! I ran 40 miles a week and that wore me out. My back's been a whole lot better since I have slowed down. About environmental factors? I don't know.

C: You're not running as much now?

S: No, I'm not running as much; I'm walking. I ran a little bit yesterday morning. I call it a "rog" now. I run and jog. I'll run for a while and then I'll stop and walk. I get to look at everything. I used to go out for 20 minutes and finish exhausted. Now I'm out for an hour and I feel great. Before, I didn't look forward to running. I'd think, "Well, I've got to run." That isn't it now. Now I walk two or three times a day.

I competed with myself and I'd try to make it in 22 minutes, if the day before I ran the same distance in 23 minutes. The next time, I'd run 15 minutes down and 15 minutes back and find a new mark. I had to run farther. I had to watch my watch. Now, it is different. We ran in the Port Townsend race that I've run in for 16 straight years. Seven-and-a-half miles, and I've never walked a second of it. It has always been flat out as hard as I could go. I ran it one year in 54 minutes, which was pretty fast. I averaged about six minutes, thirty seconds a mile. That made me feel great. The last time Linda and I walked for a while, ran for a while and walked for a while. I had never run or walked it with her before. I was always with the guys, bolting ahead and competing.

C: So cancer has changed that part of your life?

S: Yeah. I'm not that competitive anymore. Although I think part of the reason I'm surviving is because I am competitive, and I want to win. But I am much different now. I'm a walker now, not a runner.

At the last Port Townsend race I met a guy I used to run with. He finished in about an hour and five minutes. I told him I finished in an hour and twenty-five minutes and he said, "God, you're out of shape, you pig. What's wrong with you?" I told him. Now walking is just fine. I'm still adjusting to the fact that when I'm walking, and a car passes me that I'm *not* running. I have a new level of intensity and also a new level of relaxation.

C: Do you think that there was a connection with breast cancer and what was happening to you, six to eighteen months ago?

S: I've been sitting in front of a CRT (cathode ray tube/computer monitor) a lot. I don't know if that's a risk factor, but I've been doing that for 15 years. All those cathode ray tubes bombarding my chest with all that stuff. I don't know.

C: Exactly when and how was your breast cancer discovered?

S: March 8. I had a lump right underneath my nipple. It was a little knobby spot. I'd noticed it for two or three months. It didn't really get any bigger. I didn't tell anybody. It wasn't anything I was worried about. I thought it was a clogged duct or something like that. I mentioned it to Linda one night. She felt it, and said, "You need to have that looked at." Women are more sensitive to those things, I think. Lumps in breasts are big things to women, but not necessarily to men.

The next day, I saw the doctor. He said, "Well it's probably not anything, but I want you to have a mammogram today." I had a mammogram done that day—that was Monday. I picked up the results on Tuesday and made an appointment with the surgeon that day. I looked at the report in the elevator on the way up to the doctor and it said *carcinogenic!* I thought, "Oh, shit!"

When I showed it to the surgeon, he said, "Well, they're used to looking at women's breasts. This could be cancer, but there's 75 percent chance it isn't. It's tissue. It's thicker and it's showing up." He didn't think it was cancer. Well, I thought, we'll get it out and everything will be fine. He scheduled surgery for the next day. The doctor made a cut right underneath the dark part of my nipple.

C: What kind of breast cancer was it?

S: It was an estrogen receptor positive tumor, interductal. It had broken out of the ducts and invaded the surrounding tissue.

C: Into the chest wall?

S: No, for some reason, breast tissue was growing on the left side. It wasn't hormonal because I would have been growing breast tissue on both sides. So it was an anomaly. The doctor couldn't explain it. The only thing that we could think of, the only way they have ever seen that happen, is from some sort of injury. A blow could have stimulated the growth of breast tissue. There was a lump of breast tissue growing on my left side and on top of that was the tumor. Whether or not they came along together, they don't know.

C: Do you remember any injury there?

S: Well, I got elbowed a lot playing basketball, but I don't remember anything specific. The tumor spread into that breast tissue instead of the chest wall.

C: Was there lymph node involvement?

S: I had 16 lymph nodes removed, but it was a focus in just one. Whether or not it got into that one lymph node and then spread out into my system, I don't know. That's why I'm having chemo. The surgeon said it was small, 8 mm, and medium-fast growing. He said there was a good chance that it was all there was and hadn't spread to my lungs—95 percent chance. He tried to take it off and leave a margin, but it was so backed up behind my nipple that it was difficult. He wanted to leave a dime's worth of tissue underneath my nipple to provide blood flow to keep my nipple alive. But before he went back in and looked at the lymph nodes, he wanted to see if it had spread beyond that.

I had the surgery on Wednesday, and on Friday I went into Evergreen Hospital. They shot me up with this glowy stuff, and I had a bone scan. That was the scariest day of my life. I have had a lot of sport injuries, and they all showed up. Everything was glowing. I'd been having problems with my shoulder for years. They went back, tipped me on my side and scanned some more. They kept looking at it and sent the pictures down to X-ray—my thumbs, fingers, knees and my back. I have some early stages of arthritis in the middle of my back, so it really lit up in there. Then the chest X-ray. They had to redo the chest X-ray. The scan started at one o'clock and finished at six thirty.

C: All this in the same day?

S: Yes. They kept taking all these pictures. As soon as I sat down in the waiting room, they'd get me for another look.

C: Did you have somebody with you in the waiting room?

S: No. I didn't. Linda and I didn't think going for some X-rays was a big deal. I didn't realize it was going to be that traumatic. She still feels bad about not having been there.

I was sitting in the waiting room and the nurse came in and said, "Dr. Sargur (my oncologist) is just across the street. He's going to come over and see you." I thought, "Oh, shit! She can't tell me, so he's coming. I was in a sweat. I was thinking, "Oh man, this is it!" I was really worried.

Dr. Sargur came. There was one woman in the waiting room and he said, "Well, let's find another room where we can talk." I was thinking, "Oh my God! We went into a vacant X-ray room. He said, "Well, we looked at everything. You're clear." I grabbed him and hugged him and picked him up. Then I hugged the nurse. Then, I was really skeptical. I said, "Why did they take so many X-rays? " Sargur responded, "We wanted to be sure." I said, "I want to talk to the guy who read the X-rays." Sargur said I really didn't need to do that. I insisted." I want to talk to him. Let's go down to see him right now." So, we walked down the hall, and the radiologist took me through all the X-rays. I called my surgeon that night, and asked, "Now, would those guys lie to me?" I wanted a bunch of reassurance.

C: So you could buy into it?

S: That's right. So that Friday was over. Then the following Friday, the surgeon went in and took the rest of my nipple off, because he wasn't sure that he'd gotten a complete margin. As it turned out, he had gotten it all. So it really was an unnecessary surgery. I don't care. Then he went in and he took my lymph nodes out and that recovery time was pretty bad.

C: What do you mean?

S: It was hard. I had a drain in two different holes on my chest, one to the first surgery and one to the lymph node area. I had two tubes going right into my skin for two weeks. It was awful. Once the tubes came out, the fluid would build up behind the incision, because the lymph nodes weren't there to remove the fluid. It would get really thick—really uncomfortable. I couldn't put my arm down on it and I couldn't get my arm up very high. If I pulled it up, it put a lot of pressure on the whole area and stretched it out. A couple of times when I was doing my exercises the fluid just shot out. It was terrible. I thought, "God, I'm a freak." It bothered me a lot when it got so full and I would just push on the incision until "Kershwoosh!" It would fire out and hit the mirror. When it had drained, it would feel so good! I told the surgeon about it. He said I had to stop doing that because my body had to find new absorption paths. That happened slowly in about a week and a half. I finally got to the point where it wasn't draining on my clothes anymore and I didn't have to wear all the gauze. It got better. Every time I'd go to see the doctor, he'd say I wasn't able to lift my arm high enough yet.

C: You didn't have anybody from Reach to Recovery contact you about the exercises that might help your recovery?

S: My surgeon showed me. I was really careful, because I didn't want to pop the incisions. There were times when lifting my arms over my head would just about kill me. I couldn't stretch my arm up or it would pull like crazy, because everything had shortened up. Once, I was lifting my arm and I heard this big pop. BAM! I thought, what was that?" Maybe I'd broken a rib or something. One of these stringy adhesions had popped loose. My wife is a physical therapist and she helped me quite a bit. Then it was just a matter of going to Dr. Sargur and starting chemo. Now I'm half-way through chemo. I have three more months left.

C: What chemo agents are you on?

S: Methotrexate, 5 FU (Fluorouracil) and Cytoxan.

C: Does it affect your stomach?

S: I don't get really nauseous. I'm taking Zophran for nausea now, which is pretty good stuff. When I go in for my two shots on day one and day eight, I take it that day and two days following. I've been taking Zophran every once in a while when I feel that the Cytoxan is working me over. It has pretty instant effects. But I don't want to get used to it. I think it makes me more constipated.

I don't like chemotherapy. I know that people tell me that I'm doing great, but I still don't like it. Chemotherapy is having a severe effect on my immune system—my white blood cells. I go in for a blood test today. It will show me that I'm down in the I-could-be-hospitalized range because I'm susceptible to all illnesses when I'm down this far. In fact, I'm supposed to be two weeks on and two weeks off. Last month I couldn't start after the last week, because my blood count was down so far.

C: How do you think breast cancer is different for you as a man, as opposed to how it is for a woman?

S: I've kidded about it a little bit. I say every once in a while, "My body is not going to win any wet T-shirt contest anyway." A good friend of mine died of cancer when he was twenty. The cancer was in his knee. They wanted to amputate his leg and they gave him an 80 percent chance of living. He didn't do it, and he died two years later. I don't see it as a lot different from having it in my knee. If it had been on the side of my face, if I had lost an arm or a leg, where it was really visible, that would have bothered me. I'm self-conscious about it when I'm in a locker room showering. But I haven't lost a part of my identity as a result of it. I know that is not always true for women. All the breast enlargement surgeries are testimonies that women care a lot about it. It hasn't been like that for me. I guess, I feel somewhat disfigured. But there are so many other priorities in my life and one of them is living. It's much more important for me to lose 20 pounds—that's what I need to do—than to agonize over this. This is an illness; it is not a physical loss.

C: If it had been on your face—if it had been something that affected more closely, your significant identity, would your reaction to it have been different?

S: It would have. Maybe I'm not done with the gestation of those feelings. I think, initially, what you want to do is live. In five years your priorities may change. Not only do I want to live, but I want to have my breast back. Will I go in and have reconstructive surgery? Right now, I think unequivocally the answer is no. Maybe the lag time for me is much longer in the way I prioritize the negative aspect of the illness. The most important thing to me is that I live, and that I have a chance to fulfill some things I want to do with my life. To play it out within the vision I had anticipated, which was to live into my 70s or 80s and do a lot of the things that come with retirement and that part of my life. That's really important to me now. Maybe as I go along, I will loose that urgency. I think I will just make the adjustment.

For me, breast cancer is not a lot different than a heart attack or cancer in some other part of my body. I can't imagine people having cancer and not having support. It's got to be a lonely venture. I don't know what it's like for a woman to lose her breast and have that part of her identity chopped away.

C: Are you going to have radiation therapy?

S: It is my understanding that there is nothing to irradiate.

C: Is there anything you would like to pass on or say to a male who has just been diagnosed or may already be dealing with cancer?

S: I don't know. I'm ignorant enough about the woman's point of view of breast cancer that I don't see it as a male thing or a female thing.

I see it as a human issue. You know how after you buy a house, they say that you get buyer's remorse? If you know that you're going to have that, you can lessen the pain. If you send your kid away to camp, and he is gone for a week, he will experience homesickness. You discuss homesickness and you give him some ways to deal with it: "Here's a bunny rabbit, and here's a picture of mom and dad, and here's the stuff you won't care about for the first three or four days, but maybe that fifth day it will mean a little bit more to you and help sustain you."

I think there are some markers. It would have helped me to know that I was going to have a couple of months of depression. One of the things that happens to some people is that closing down, that cocooning. It's a way to protect yourself, but the sooner you acknowledge that and get on with the job of living, the sooner you'll be able to stimulate whatever connection you have with your immune system. I felt better with chemotherapy each month rather than worse. Not only do I have confidence that I can get through this, but I'm also confident that I'm not going to be "whacked out." I think that my own immune system is recovering faster because I'm acknowledging happy things and use creative visualization. I'm trying to be a part of the process rather than just tagging along. Regardless of being male or female, it would have helped me to know I had options.

Dr. Mukund Sargur

Oncology, Hematology, Internal Medicine
Evergreen Hospital, Kirkland, WA
Taped Interview June 19, l989, updated January 1995

A Brief History

Clo: Could you give us an overview of the treatment of breast cancer?

Dr. Sargur: Breast cancer has been around as long as people. But the treatment of cancer has radically changed, especially in the last 15 to 20 years. All cancers are approached with three methods: one is surgery, the second is radiation, and the third is drugs. Surgery has been here the longest. When there is a lump, or any mass in the body, the instinct is to cut it out. The "old" theory was that the more tumor you removed, the more tissue you removed, the more cancer you had taken out.

The first breast cancer surgery, devised by Halsted at the turn of the century, consisted of the surgeon taking the breast, the muscles—he took everything out. The end result was that the patient and the family could be assured that most of the affected tissue was taken away—however, it left behind a very disfigured human being. At that time plastic surgery was not very developed. Interestingly, many of these patients ended up with the cancer coming back.

C: So, in the end, it didn't get rid of the problem?

S: No. After the surgery, the doctor would go to the patient's room and say, "I'm happy to tell you that I got it all." For the patient it is a great feeling that it's all gone.

[Then, at times] the tumor would come back in the armpits, and the doctor would say, "Maybe we should be taking out more area. We should be doing something with lymph nodes."

Then doctors started adding radiation treatment to the armpit. This was a British technique. It was called McQuitter's Technique. McQuitter was a Scottish radiation therapist.

But remember, the theory we are dealing with is that cancer creeps along on foot—meaning, it started in the breast, then it went to the armpit, then, if left alone for some more time, it goes into the rest of your body. The surgeon took care of the breast cancer, and the radiation therapy burned it in the next field, because, after all, how much more can you grab from the armpit and pull out? Technically, it is not possible. There are delicate structures, and blood vessels and nerves involved. So, the surgeon [performed the surgery], then, handed the patient over to the radiation therapist who proceeded with the next area of battle.

C: Did the cancer normally go back into the lymph nodes, or did it go into the muscle underneath the armpit?

S: Both. If the tumor is large enough, it can invade the muscle directly. That's why doctors literally scraped it off the chest wall, leaving nothing but bare wall. And, it may have penetrated through the chest wall muscle, which is when they would cut up a part of the chest wall and put in some prosthesis. Technically, it could be done when the therapy was available. And, they did the same thing with the armpit, cutting as much as possible. But the cancer is still going right into your chest. There is no stopping cancer just because your anatomy acts as if it could stop it. That's only the extent of the reach of the surgeon from the outside.

Of course, if [the cancer] came back, the surgeon felt that maybe he didn't go far enough—but couldn't technically. So, he asked the radiologist to take over with radiation treatment. An X-ray beam can be directed anywhere.

The patients ended up with swollen arms [lymphedema], because the radiation destroyed all the lymphatics. The doctor took out as much as possible, [and the radiologist took care of the lymphatics], but the end result was a human being who was mutilated to a large extent. Still, [the patient's] greatest hope was that they got all the cancer. But most of the recurrences, or relapses, were not local: they were distant—the liver, the lung, the brain or the bones.

C: So the cancer would still continue to travel?

S: Right. That was the time that theory changed; [we recognized] that breast cancer is not a LOCAL disease, but a SYSTEMIC disease—a very important concept.

C: Intriguing! That must be why there is such a main-enance problem.

S: You got it. The whole concept was that cancer was a surgical disease at the turn of the century, and then things were turned around by our statistics. It is not the tumor that kills the patient: it's the spreading of the disease.

C: When did the theory change from surgical to systemic?

S: I would say in the late '60s, or early '70s. Now that the shift emphasis changed to all over the body, the surgeon could confidently say, "All I'm going to take out is the little cancer," and not feel bad that he didn't get it all.

Radiation therapy is the initial background of armpit [therapy]. The patients ended up with swollen arms—non-functional, terrible arms. And still, the cancer returned. That's when the therapy was totally dropped.

Bonnadona, a surgeon from Italy, came up with the theory that you don't even have to remove the breast. All you have to do is take out the lump, then apply radiation to the surrounding breast area. If microscopic spots show up, then burn them off, so that the patient has a functional body—nothing artificial. The woman retains her breast.

Then there is the problem of women with small breasts. If you take out a big chunk of breast tissue in a small-breasted person, you end up disfiguring it anyway. So, [it was decided to] take out the entire breast, rather than leave half of it. Sometimes, some of the chemotherapy drugs we use along with radiation can have a reaction on the breast, and a woman can end up with a shriveled, scarred-up breast.

C: Then, part of the adjunct therapy, not only the surgery, might deform the breast?

S: Right.

C: Is that due primarily to chemotherapy ?

S: And radiation—a combination. So, [it was thought] maybe we should not treat the patients with both concurrently. Maybe, they should be given sequentially—drugs first, then radiation, so there's no interaction between the two.

STAGES OF BREAST CANCER

The first thing I need to do [as an oncologist], from my perspective, is to see what stage you are in; meaning, the early stage, or the more advanced stage, [in order to] treat the breast cancer. A study was done to determine the stages. [The researchers] have divided all breast cancer patients [into those] stages.

Stage 1 is when the breast cancer is only in the breast.

Stage 2 is when it's in the lymph nodes.

Stage 3-A is when lots of lymph nodes are involved

Stage 3-B is when even more lymph nodes are involved, and the tumor is sort of stuck to the surrounding area in the armpit.

Stage 4 is to find it extended (metastasized).

Let us say we are now dealing with Stage 1, Stage 2 and Stage 3-A patients. We think additional therapy at this stage will make a difference in the long run. If we find someone in Stage 4 at the beginning of treatment, it's hard for them to survive. It would be ideal, of course, to catch someone in Stage 1, so that the surgery and the radiation therapy get rid of the tumor completely.

C: Have you noticed any patterns with the patients with whom you've dealt in Stage 1—any patterns in their lives, other than the medical ones—that might make a difference in their recovery?

S: That's a very tough thing to quantify. All I can quantify are medical facts. How do you quantify emotions? How do you quantify the inherent biology of the person? It figures in the resistance. There are some people who are very good at 80 years of age. They are still very functional, while 70-year-olds are confined to wheelchairs. It's incredible.

And, you wonder why? Here are two human beings born with the same potential. Did they inherit some defective genes? Or is it something they did to their bodies? These are philosophical, as well as physiological, questions. I can look at a piece of breast tissue under a microscope, and tell you exactly what it's going to do—to the best of my present knowledge.

Let's say we have a Stage 1 breast cancer. The first thing we do is measure the size of the tumor. Next, we take sections of the tumor, and stain it with dyes—blue and pink dyes. We look at the tumor under the microscope—they produce very colorful images. In fact, my major hobby is art. I do a lot of painting and I get ideas when I look at tumors.

C: Remarkable.

S: They're bizarre. They're beautiful. They're proliferating, bursting forth, aggressive, groping. They are especially colorful with leukemia. There's a doctor by the name of Quigliado, a British hematologist. When you go through Quigliado's book of leukemia, it's like going through *Life* magazine. All those colorful pictures.

C: Is that because different kinds of tissues pick up different colors?

S: Exactly. Each tumor has a tendency to pick up a different color, or [has] a different method of picking it up. A pathologist depends entirely on morphology [the study of form and structure of organisms] to make a diagnosis. It's the structure of the tumor [that's important to him]. The surgeon goes by his feel, like, Dr. Lennard says, "It doesn't feel right. It's very tough, gritty, firm." These are the words used for texture and feel. But, the pathologist is all visual. He can never touch the slides. They are all cut and made into a two-dimensional object from a three-dimensional object. Of course, when he gets a specimen, he does have the opportunity to look at it and make slides, cut it open, take a magnifying glass and look inside. When he looks into the microscope, that's the time he sees all the pattern of the tumor, and he looks at what it does to the normal tissue. They take a section on the edge of the tumor, never from the middle.

C: Why is that?

S: [The pathologist] needs to see what the tumor is doing at the edge. How it is reacting, progressing. At the edge you can look for infiltration—whether it has invaded blood vessels, whether it has broadened into the lymphatics, and you look at the differentiation.

Differentiation means that when you look at normal breast tissue it will have a nice, uniform structure. It will have ducts. The breast is a gland; it is [partially made up of] sacs. Breast cancer [usually] develops from the duct, the lining of the tube that brings the milk. It is an infiltrating ductal carcinoma. If you look at [the pathologist's] report, that is how he describes it. So, if the cancer mimics the original breast tissue, then it's in a well-differentiated shape. Meaning, as the tissues grow, they have a tendency to mimic where they came from.

That's why—if the breast cancer spreads to the brain, and you take a section of the brain—the pathologist will tell you, "This looks like breast cancer." He will not tell you it is brain cancer, because he is so used to looking at the breast and breast tissue, he knows how it looks. He knows it is out of place in the brain. He doesn't call it brain cancer.

C: It really LOOKS like the breast cancer?

S: Yes, it does!

C: Amazing! You'd think it would take on the characteristics of the brain tissue.

S: But it doesn't do that. For instance, if liver cancer goes to the brain, it looks like the liver in the brain!

C: Remarkable!

S: Yes. Each organ has a [unique] pattern.

BREAST CANCER: A SYSTEMIC DISEASE

C: Is that how they discovered that cancer is systemic, because they could identify that pattern throughout the body?

S: Yes.

C: What about the spread of breast cancer?

S: It depends on the aggressiveness of the tumor. Axillary lymph node status is the critical issue in predicting survival. If cancer is found in the lymph nodes, it is telling you that it's the kind that spreads, or that it's gone from here to there, and has gotten into some important road-ways, which are lymphatic channels, and possibly the blood stream. It gives us a clue.

Originally, [doctors] thought that if they found the lymph nodes positive, the tumor had gone from here to there, and had stopped there. So, if they removed it, they got rid of it. But we have discovered since then that these are footprints of what's happened beyond. So that information is only giving you news.

C: Of what's potentially going on elsewhere?

S: That's right.

C: But you mentioned different types of breast cancers. Are there types of breast cancers which do not transfer? Or, do all types transfer to different areas of the body?

S: That's a very good question. There are some cancers which grow locally, maybe to a big size, but still when we look at them, we know that these are not the type that spread.

C: So you can tell under the microscope?

S: That's what the path report is going for. They are looking for whether the cancer is a locally aggressive tumor which seldom metastasizes, like medullary carcinoma, or whether it might be infiltrating ductal carcinoma, which does typically metastasize, or, perhaps, inflammatory breast cancer—even if it's tiny, you know it's all over the body. Inflammatory breast cancer usually occurs in young women. It looks like an infection—redness, tenderness—but when you try to drain the abscess, no pus comes out.

STATISTICS

C: What about breast cancer survival statistics?

S: The 5- or 10-year breast cancer numbers represent a statistical analysis. A lot of people misunderstand *the meaning* of the five years and ten years. I told one patient that she had a 50 percent chance of surviving five years, and she broke down. "If I only have five years, why should I bother to talk with you?" she asked.

I said, "I'm not telling you that you're going to live for five years. At five years, the statistics were analyzed, and they found that 50 percent of the patients were alive. If you are part of that 50 percent you may live forever!" But the analysis was done in five years, because when a study is done we must stop and say, okay, in five years, how many are alive?

If you look at Stage 1 breast cancer, 85 percent of the patients are alive in five years. But, the other 15 percent [even] in Stage 1, did not make it to five years. If there is only one percent that did not make it, and that one percent is you, it is 100 percent failure for you.

C: So true.

S: Statistics are a big nuisance for the patients and the doctors. For a global understanding of the disease in a non-emotional, scientific way, they're great. You can throw out numbers, and then, forget it.

C: But, not in terms of people.

S: Not in terms of people. The prognosis worsens as the number of lymph nodes increases.

PATHOLOGY

S: Next—the histopathology. I told you about differentiation, remember? Differentiated means it can mimic the original tumor. But, some tumors grow so rapidly, that they don't have time to mimic the parent, or where they came from. It's called a poorly differentiated tumor. The pathologist's nightmare is to work with a poorly-differentiated tumor. You remove the tumor, and it looks like a sheet of malignant cells. You say, "Hey, Joe, what do you think? Where did it come from?" He'll say, "I don't know. It is poorly-differentiated. It could be the lung, it could be the liver, it could be the breast." Its origin cannot be identified because the tumor hasn't taken time to mimic its parent. The tumor has grown so rapidly, that it's just...growing. In order to form a tumor that looks like its original, it takes time to build the structures, the ducts, and the tubes, and so forth.

C: So, in my particular case, it was well-differentiated?

S: Yes.

C: Which indicated that it was slow-growing?

S: That's correct. Your tumor was a "good boy." It took its time to grow! [laughter] Histopathology is a very important aspect. The poorly differentiated tumor is the worst prognosis, the well-differentiated is the best, and then, there are intermediate grades.

S: There is also the lymphocytic infiltration of the tumor. Lymphocytes are the cells that give you immunity to fight infections. We can actually see the lymphocytes attacking the tumor cells in the tissue. There is a host-tumor relationship already established. We really don't know the ultimate significance of everything, but we see all these patterns when we look at the tumors.

Another important factor is the presence of the estrogen and progesterone receptors. When you still have ovaries, during the monthly cycle, the breasts get tender, because there are switches, or receptors, on top of the breast cells. The female hormone flows into the switch, turns it on, and helps the breast do its function.

The female hormone helps the cancer grow—the estrogen adds fuel to the fire. If the cancer cells have lots of receptors, it means that they, the tumor, took the time to build those receptors. That makes it a slow-growing tumor.

C: It sounds like a two-edged sword.

S: It *is* a two-edged sword. If you have lots of receptors in the tumor, it's a good sign, because the tumor took time to grow. If it's a poorly-differentiated tumor, it has hardly any receptors, because it grew so rapidly. The advantage of the tumor with many receptors is that you have something to turn it off with.

MEDICAL STUDIES

S: There are different phases [to be aware of] in a medical study.

Phase 1 studies in cancer try to find out how much [medication] a patient can take.

Phase 2 studies [discover] how much medication a physician can give, and what side effects can be seen.

Phase 3 studies compare [the new treatment] with standard treatment.

C: I see what you're saying. When we hear a drug is safe, it might still be in the first phase. That would explain why all of a sudden we might hear about its side effects.

S: Exactly.

C: Are these studies done by FDA?

S: Yes. Like Laetrile. The people in Mexico accused the United States government of not using their drug, because it was "highly successful." There was so much public pressure on the our government to test the drug. "This is a miracle drug," they said. People were going across the border and buying it in bushels, spending millions of dollars on this "miracle drug." Finally the United States tested it in a scientific pattern, and found it to be absolutely useless!

ADDITIONAL DIAGNOSTIC FACTORS

S: Then, there's one last factor. It's called the "Proliferative Index," which is nothing more than looking at the DNA itself. Pathologists take the tumor and mash it up, and make it into a solution—actual DNA content of each tumor cell. If there is a lot of DNA in a cancer cell, it's nothing but a blueprint for growth. It means it's an aggressive tumor. Normally, the DNA content is divided between the two parents. Your mom gave you some, and your dad gave you some. So, there are two sets of chromosomes. All these cancer cells have three sets. It's like a three-headed monster!

There's too much DNA. When they began to multiply, they acquired from other cells, or they multiplied some other way. They have the potential for growth, with all kinds of chromosomes—very disorganized.

The normal growth in the body is under highly scientific direction by the nucleus. As soon as it reaches a certain size, it says, "Stop"—and, it stops growing. But, cancer has none of these growth-stopping codes in it. Researchers are interested in finding out more about the DNA. They have discovered a gene that controls breast cancer. The gene is called "HER-2neu." If we can switch off this abnormal gene in the body, maybe that's the way to cure cancer—if there is some way we can turn it off. It would be like a vaccination for cancer. I don't know if we will be able to do it, but that's the way we are heading.

We are acquiring more and more knowledge about the human body. In fact, the Human Genome Project is the most expensive, and biggest project ever undertaken on by the United States health industry.

C: That's the DNA project you're talking about?

S: Yes. The project is headed by Watson—Watson & Crick—British scientists who cracked the DNA mystery in 1951. The two scientists photographed DNA for the first time. It's called the coil of life. The chromosome can be stretched out for miles, and each spot is occupied by a gene, and each gene has a function in the body. Each gene is supposed to make a hormone, or an enzyme, or an acid, or something for its growth. There is a process of analyzing each gene, and that information is being fed into a computer for storage—billions and billions of pieces of data. (*See also* Causes of Breast Cancer: Genetic Factors.)

THE FUTURE

S: Let's say Clo comes to me in the year 2020. I take a piece of her skin, mash it up, and put it into a data machine. It will give me a genetic code on her. I'll say, "Clo is high risk for breast cancer, because she's got the 'HER-2neu' gene sitting around. She's high risk for colon cancer, and she's high risk for this or that." It will give me a readout.

C: Then, you will know specifically what to do instead of having to guess.

S: I hope so. But, this might make a patient so nervous that she doesn't want to live. Do you know what I mean? If she knows all the risks? Knowledge is strange. Sometimes too much knowledge is not good.

HOPE

C: With your knowledge as an oncologist, it must be difficult for you when a patient comes in with a Stage 4 cancer. How do you deal with that without dashing all hope?

S: It is very difficult. That is when philosophy comes in. That is where religion comes in. That is where a sense of humor comes in. All are crutches we hang on to dearly. Without a sense of humor, my goodness, you can't do it! Let's say that the surgeon has had a go at it, radiation therapists have had a go at it, and now, something more is needed. It is a systemic disease. That is the most important concept to get into. It is a disease which has spread all over the body from day one. (That's if it's in Stage 4.)

We need to treat the patient with drugs. Unfortunately, the drugs we have are like hitting someone with a sledge hammer. It attacks anything that grows in the body. So, we need to get a Therapeutic Index—meaning, *the drug should kill more cancer cells than healthy body tissue,* so that the end result is: more cancer is gone, and some normal tissue remain. A drug is considered extremely safe if the Therapeutic Index is *wide,* but if the Therapeutic Index is *narrow,* then we have to deal in very minute doses. We can't go beyond that dosage, because it could kill too many good cells.

We calculate all the dosages based on body weight, and body surface area.

CHEMOTHERAPY AND TAMOXIFEN

C: Do patients usually lose their hair with chemotherapy?

S: Not necessarily. There are some drugs that cause hair loss and others that don't.

C: Does chemotherapy have an effect on breast cancer survival rates?

S: Exactly. We have improved them by 20 percent. In cancer, a killer disease that affects so many women, that 20 percent translates into thousands of lives saved.

S: Let's talk about the risk factors. Who should get these treatments, and who should not? Should we subject everyone to chemotherapy who has breast cancer, or only a select few?

We started out saying that for Stage 2 people with breast cancer, the tumor has spread to the lymph nodes. In Stage 1, 15 percent of the people do not make it as far as five years. We need to recognize— though we call them Stage 1—we might have missed something:

1) Maybe we didn't examine enough lymph nodes;

2) Maybe it had gotten right into the chest wall; or

3) The tumor didn't get into the lymphatics, but maybe it is so aggressive that it just went right into the blood stream.

In that case, we are understaging this patient. We're telling her it is Stage 1, when it is truly Stage 2, and she should be getting treatment. This aspect of the controversy is being examined, and we are beginning to treat even Stage 1 breast cancer with chemotherapy.

C: Which is why you offered to me tamoxifen chemotherapy?

S: Right. Because you fit into the hardest group. I need to look at what the factors in that group are. They are:
- If the estrogen/progesterone receptors are negative;
- If you have a poorly differentiated tumor; and
- If you have more than two chromosomes in your DNA.

INCREASED RISK FACTORS FOR BREAST CANCER

Here is a list of factors associated with increased risk for record of disease:
- If the lymph nodes are positive.
- If the estrogen/progesterone status is negative.
- If the tumor size is over 5 cm.
- If the tissue has high nuclear grade (if the nucleus of the cancer cell looks very different from the nucleus of a normal cell).
- If the DNA content shows aneuploidy (abnormality of DNA).
- If there is a high "S" factor (number of cells in the "synthesis phase" of the cell cycle—preparing to divide).
- If gene p53 or gene BRCA1, located on Chromosome 17, are found to be mutated (abnormal).
- If tumor angiogenesis, microblood vessels developed to support the growth of the tumor, is present.

C: In my case, would you say: that I am high-risk, or low-risk?

S: Let's go back in your records. Here's your DNA content. It can be seen by the little aneuploid peak—there are a few cells in your case which are bad. Secondly, your estrogen/progesterone receptors are positive. And, here's your pathology report: Tumor is measured 3.5 cm. Moderate nuclear grade, regular infiltrating, 14 lymph nodes negative. Here is the only thing: it was a slight aneuploid. So, if we give you marks, we can say—we can call it either way.

C: There's a possibility, but you don't really know whether the cancer will come back?

S: Yes, that's why I was wondering whether to give you chemo or not—because of all of the things I was weighing. Since the tamoxifen can force it down, should we go at it with a little "bang" of drugs, and see if we can get rid of some cancer cells that may be lurking around, and then put you on a long-term tamoxifen? Since the study is not done on Stage 1, I can't recommend that with full confidence. Maybe five years from now, we may be treating everybody with chemotherapy. I don't know.

TREATMENT

C: Let's shift for a moment, if you don't mind. What significant factors support the choice for a patient between a *modified radical mastectomy* (MRM) and a *lumpectomy with radiation therapy* (RT)?

S: The choice depends on the
- size of tumor (maximum 4-5 cm)
- size of the breast
- location of the tumor

The surgeon should be able to excise the tumor with healthy margins and still be able to preserve a cosmetically aesthetic breast for the choice to be lumpectomy with radiation therapy.

The ultimate outcome for both mastectomy, and lumpectomy with radiation are the same. The advantages and disadvantages of each are listed below:

	ADVANTAGES	*DISADVANTAGES*
MASTECTOMY	No need for radiation therapy No need for further mammograms	Loss of breast Need for reconstruction

LUMPECTOMY
+ RADIATION
	Keep breast
	No need for reconstruction
		Need for radiation
		  therapy (5-6 weeks)
		Risk of local recurrence
		Need for further
		  mammograms
		May have lumpy breast
		  after radiation therapy

C: Which patients are considered candidates for *postoperative adjuvant chemotherapy* and/or *hormone therapy*?

S: This is a difficult question to answer. Initial studies from the last 15 years have demonstrated the benefit of adjuvant therapy in preventing and/or delaying the recurrence of breast cancer in premenopausal, lymph-node-positive women. There is also an overall improvement in survival.

More recently, postoperative chemotherapy and hormonal therapy has shown benefit in both premenopausal and postmenopausal women, with both positive and negative lymph nodes. The choice of treatment depends on:

- aggressiveness of the tumor
- receptor status
- clinical state of the patient(physical)
- flow cytometry data

Tamoxifen (anti-estrogen hormone) has been shown to improve disease-free survival and overall survival. This is good news. Plus, the combination of chemotherapy and tamoxifen therapy are currently being studied. Early results suggest a significant benefit from the combination of this treatment.

C: What are the advantages and disadvantages of hormone therapy?

S: The benefits from hormonal treatment include:

- A decrease of new breast cancer in the opposite breast by 50 percent.
- Prevention of calcium loss from bones (osteoporosis).
- Improvement in the lipid profile (cholesterol).
- The inducement of vaginal secretions for lubrication in post-menopausal women.
- A decrease in the incidence of ovarian cancer by 50 percent.

S: The disadvantages of tamoxifen therapy are:

- It causes an increase in the severity of hot flashes.
- Menstrual irregularity can occur in premenopausal women.

- An increased incidence of endometrial (lining of the uterus) cancer.
- An increased incidence of thrombophlebitis (blood clot and inflammation of a vein, often occurring in the legs).
- Depression in 1-10 percent of patients.
- Retinal (eye) changes in rare cases, usually reversible.
- Increased estrogens in premenopausal women which can cause PMS-like symptoms.
- Costs $75-$80 per month.

C: When is a patient considered for radiation therapy following a mastectomy?

S: A patient would be considered a candidate for radiation therapy when there is:

- A large tumor (greater than 5 cm).
- Any skin involvement.
- The cancer is inflammatory carcinoma.
- There are more than four lymph nodes involved.
- There is a spread of cancer through the capsule of the lymph node.
- Positive surgical margins (cancer cells still detected in tissues surrounding the surgical site) are detected by the pathologist.

C: What is inflammatory breast cancer, and how should it be treated?

S: Inflammatory breast cancer is a virulent (highly malignant) form of breast cancer which can rapidly spread to the rest of the body. It is very aggressive.

The first treatment for inflammatory breast cancer is chemotherapy. Once the disease is controlled, local surgery or radiation therapy is given to control the tumor. This is again followed by more chemotherapy. Bone marrow transplantation is an experimental form of treatment being tried. The 5 year survival has been improved to 50-60 percent.

C: Are women with breast cancer prone to other cancers?

S: Yes. Colon cancer and ovarian cancer has been linked to women with breast cancer.

C: Do men get breast cancer?

S: Yes. It is typically more aggressive than women's breast cancer, and more advanced when found because of the ease with which it spreads. The treatment is the same as for women: surgery, chemotherapy, and hormonal therapy.

BEING A CANCER DOCTOR

C: Dr. Sargur, why did you choose to become an oncologist?

S: All through my medical career, each specialty fascinated me so much, that I wanted to become that. I would go to my surgical rotation, and say, "Ah, this is what I must do for the rest of my life!" Then, I would get into pathology—the science of the tumor—and how it looks under the microscope. I wanted to be a pathologist. Then, I would go into internal medicine, struggling with lab tests, and I would say, "Oh, I must be an internist." It's like Sherlock Holmes, you know? And then, I would see patients in the grips of emotions—parents dying, or children dying, and—you know what? The mind's the most powerful organ in our bodies because, without our brain, we're dead, even if our organs are all functioning. What really matters is the mind. I almost signed up to be a psychiatrist at one time. But then, I said to myself, if I become a psychiatrist, I will lose all the skills I have acquired as a medical student.

I asked myself, which field can encompass all of these specialties? It was oncology. I deal with the tumor, sometimes I do surgery—I take out a little bit of lump and send it to the lab. Medicine is involved, because I prescribe drugs. And, I'm dealing with the mind all the time.

C: Do you have a sense of what is causing the increasing number of cancer patients?

S: It's a tough question, because we have to look at the trend over decades. Technology is changing so rapidly. What your grandmother died of was [what they called] a stroke. For all you know, it might have been breast cancer fifty years ago.

Now that we have the breast under the microscope, literally, with mammograms, and figuratively, with public awareness. It may appear the trend is increasing, when it may be just that we are dealing with more and more of it.

C: What do you see for the future of cancer, in terms of cures and in terms of handling the disease?

S: For one thing we're trying to prevent cancer. It's like smallpox—eradicate it 100 percent. If we can identify the people at high risk, screen them, and see if we can get it at an earlier stage. We may change our dietary habits, and we could find what factors are involved with cancer, and change them. We may be intricately involved with cancer, because our life style may be carcinogenic, and we may have to give up certain things that we do right now.

C: You mean, change our life style?

S: Change our life style, if we want freedom from cancer as the ultimate goal. But the life in the fast lane may be so exciting that we may rather have cancer than give that up. It's like cocaine, or like any other addiction.

C: What patterns have you observed in your patients that through the years have enabled them to be among the survivors in the statistics?

S: All I have told you so far has been highly supported by data, but there's always the one anecdotal patient who was supposed to do badly, who doesn't, and does get better. So, medicine is still an art. Though we put on the garb of scientist, there is still an unknown factor, and we're all in search of that unknown factor. Until that is nailed down, I can, for that reason alone, never take away hope from my cancer patients. I never say that "You are going to, or are supposed to die."

C: How do you handle dealing with so many cancer patients?

S: I look at it as somebody I can hold hands with, with and take them along. I come from an Eastern philosophy (India), and Eastern philosophers believe that we are all destined to do our bit in this life and everything is preordained. It is your part to do your bit in this life. And, if you realize that, you realize there is only one "Clo" on this earth, and she is a totally unique person. There is nobody who can replace you in your physical and emotional frame of mind.

That's how I retain my identity, and work. We are not seeking *outside* for what we really are. That's where the Eastern philosophy comes in. It is not what you perceive on the outside that makes you. It is the inner self, or the happiness, that really matters.

C: That is how you are able to maintain your own inner balance in spite of all the suffering you see?

S: Yes. If we could get each of our cancer patients, to accept that concept, there would much more meaning for them—even day-to-day, even if they are destined to die in ten days—they are called to do a good job in those ten days. All of us are all running on a fuse that's burning.

C: Just becoming aware of that may enable us to live better.

S: Yes. So, if somebody has only four months to live, he better hurry up, and have a good time.

C: So, it's important for us to connect to who we really are.

S: Yes! There's no point in moping about, and feeling bad about it. Of course, the human body is important, but the SPIRIT, which cannot be touched by cancer, is the most important thing in life. You can't radiate it, you can't give it chemotherapy, believe me!

The spirit is so powerful, and all of us have that within ourselves. But, it is proportionally covered by our personality. There are quirks. So, the more you cover up your inner spirit, the less you will be able to shine, and help.

C: Thank you, Dr. Sargur, for sharing your knowledge of breast cancer with us. It will be a valuable reference for those of us with breast cancer, and for our families and friends.

"We have been through painful surgery, months of needles, toxic drugs, nausea, fatigue, low blood counts, delays in treatment, depression, hot flashes and much more. And always on our minds are the questions will it be enough, will the treatment work?"

— Linda Fankhauser, breast cancer survivor

"Lighten up. Cancer is serious, but not the end of the world! Deal with it!"

— Valerie Jean, breast cancer survivor

Stealing the Dragon's Fire
Clo Wilson-Hashiguchi

Part III:
Breast Cancer Handbook

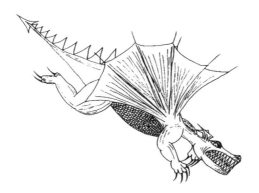

Table of Contents

NOTE: *Along with a selected bibliography, there is extensive referencing in the text of the Breast Cancer Handbook. Each major section has its **Sources** at its end. In addition, there are **Sources** listed after many of the sub-sections. Sources are indicated in the text by a number in parentheses, without an intervening space, at the end of the quotation or sentence.*

"There is a new diagnosis of Breast Cancer every 3 minutes. There is another death from Breast Cancer every 12 minutes."
— American Cancer Society

INTRODUCTION TO BREAST CANCER

The numbers are numbing. In the United States alone, according to the American Cancer Society, 182,000 women will be diagnosed with breast cancer this year, and of those 46,000 are predicted to die. 1,000 men, also, it is suggested, will be diagnosed with breast cancer, and of those, 300 are expected to die; it is a nightmare. For every person diagnosed with breast cancer, and for loved ones who become aware of the staggering numbers who deal with this disease, there are piercing questions to ask.

Why is there not more known about the prevention of breast cancer? What causes it? How can we cure it? It is the scariest thing to receive the shock of diagnosis, followed by the disillusionment that comes with realizing that the medical and scientific communities are stumped about how to cure breast cancer effectively, despite the extensive research going on.

There is progress being made in research, but it is woefully slow for the numbers of breast cancer patients coming in—mothers, daughters, sisters, grandmothers, friends and coworkers, fathers, brothers, and uncles—people who are having to deal with the disease on a daily basis. It's rather like placing a few sandbags against a flooding river, hoping to stem the flow.

WHAT IS BREAST CANCER?

It is important, first, to understand the nature of breast cancer. It is not just one disease found in the breast, but, according to the National Cancer Institute, about 20 distinctly different diseases, all different, except for two significant characteristics: 1) cancer cells grow and multiply out of control, and 2) cancer cells have the ability to travel elsewhere in the body to lodge and develop a new tumorous mass.

Healthy cells have built-in controls. They only multiply to a size that is necessary for a particular function, with great respect for the sizes and shapes the other body parts surrounding them need to function well. Not so with cancer cells. They care only about their own growth and development, and multiply until they have crowded out or made dysfunctional surrounding body parts, even to the point of closing down the whole body's functioning. The cancer cells individually are weakened cells, but together become a force to contend with.

The ability of cancer cells to travel elsewhere through the blood and lymphatic systems of the body signals that what we are dealing with is a systemic disease, not a local disease that can be cured by cutting out a local tumor and being done with it. "The tumor does not kill the patient, the metastasis (the spread) does," Dr. Mukund Sargur, Oncologist, asserts. This is why adjunct therapy—chemotherapy, hormone therapy, and/or radiation therapy—is recommended. The first two therapies are systemic in nature, attempting to ferret out all wandering cancer cells and kill them or arrest their growth before they lodge in another location and begin to create another mass. Radiation, a local therapy, attempts to kill cancer cells locally before they spread elsewhere. The fact that there are about 20 different types of breast cancer, each with their own peculiarities, offers a complex challenge to the medical and scientific communities. And, according to the National Cancer Institute, the 20 breast cancers are just a few of the over 100 cancer types (some sources say as high as 200) of cancer found in all parts of the body. Fighting cancer is learning to fight many different foes.

THE BREAST

The breast is a gland, the mammary gland, designed by nature to produce milk so that a woman can feed her infant.(1)

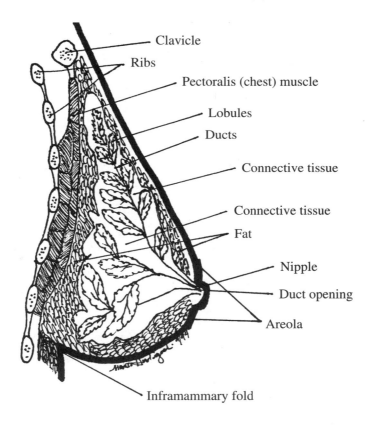

Women's breasts are many different shapes and sizes, which has no bearing on how much milk is available to an infant, or a woman's risk of getting breast cancer. As women age, their breasts which were "firmer and more conical shaped"(1) as young women, become softer, and more flat to the chest. The breast itself is composed of about one-third fat cells, the rest of breast tissue. "The fat can vary as you gain or lose weight; the breast tissue remains constant."(2) As a woman ages, the breast tissue is replaced by fat, since it is no longer needed for milk production.

Breast tissue is composed of acini, lobules, lobes, and ducts. "Acini are sacs lined with cells that can produce milk. The acini cluster together to form structures called lobules."(1) A group of lobules, called a lobe, then empties into a tube called a duct, which then extends to the nipple, where the infant can then access the milk.

Slightly below the center of the breast lie the nipple and areola, which can vary significantly in shape and color from one woman to another. The nipple becomes erect when stimulated, which allows the infant a place from which it can suck milk. The areola color varies according to the complexion. "In blondes it tends to be pink; in brunettes it's browner, and in black-skinned people, it's black."(2) The areola's color darkens with pregnancy.

BENIGN BREAST DISEASE (FIBROCYSTIC BREASTS)

Fibrocystic disease has been a catch-all medical term used to describe abnormalities in the breast which are not cancer. Abnormalities can be caused by a number of things. Dr. Susan Love places non-cancerous breast irregularities in six categories:(2)

1) Normal physiological changes (e.g., minor tenderness, swelling, and lumpiness experienced by most women during or before periods).
2) Mastalgia (severe breast pain, cyclical or noncyclical that interferes with a woman's normal life).
3) Infections and inflammations.
4) Discharge and other nipple problems.
5) Lumpiness or nodularity (greater than the norm).
6) Dominant lumps, such as cysts or fibroadenomas.

NOTE: *The presence of "atypical hyperplasia" combined with a family history of breast cancer is the only abnormal noncancerous breast condition that has been found to indicate an increased risk of breast cancer for women.*

For a more detailed listing, call the National Cancer Institute at 1-800-4-CANCER.

Sources: (1) *Breast Cancer,* by Yashar Hirshaut, M.D., F.A.C.P. and Peter I. Pressman, M.D., F.A.C.S.; (2) *Dr. Susan Love's Breast Book,* by Susan M. Love, M.D.

TYPES OF BREAST CANCER

Infiltrating/Invasive Ductal Carcinoma, cancer found in the breast ducts, is the most common type of breast cancer in women, comprising about 70-80% of all breast cancers diagnosed.

Lobular Carcinoma, cancer found in the lobules of the breast, is the breast cancer most frequently found in both breasts.

Inflammatory Carcinoma, is a very aggressive cancer, which creates a noticeable inflammation (red appearance and warmth) of the breast tissue.

Cystosarcoma Phylloides is a rare type of breast cancer normally treated with a wide incision (a wide surgical removal of the mass).

Paget's Disease is a breast cancer of the nipple, characterized by a leakage from the nipple and, at times, a tumor mass located in the ducts.

Within ductal breast cancer can be found many sub-types: intraductal in situ ("in situ" is when the cancer is not invasive), invasive, comedo, inflammatory, medullary, mucinous, papillary, scirrhous, tubular, and others. Lobular breast cancer has basically two sub-types: in situ, and invasive. Paget's Disease, a type of nipple breast cancer, includes largely two sub-types: intraductal and invasive ductal. Cytosarcoma phylloides and inflammatory carcinoma are listed by the National Cancer Institute under types of nipple breast cancer with no sub-types noted.(1)

Sources: (1) "Breast Cancer," *PDQ Information,* National Cancer Institute #208/00013, 8/1/94, 10/31/94; (2) "Cancer and Health Care Reform: NCCS Principles," National Coalition for Cancer Survivorship, May 1994; (3) "Treatment of Early-Stage Breast Cancer," National Institutes of Health Consensus Development Conference Statement, 1990.

Interview Excerpt: Dr. Mukund Sargur

C: What are "precancer" and "carcinoma in situ"?

S: Carcinoma in situ is a pathological diagnosis, which accounts for 15-20 percent of breast cancers currently being diagnosed. When a breast is biopsied, the epithelial lining of the breast ducts (DCIS), or breast lobules (LCIS) are diagnosed abnormal. DCIS and atypical hyperplasia *(see* Benign Breast Disease) are considered "precancerous" conditions, while LCIS is considered a "marker for subsequent development of invasive disease, rather than a premalignant lesion."(2)

Lobular carcinoma in situ (LCIS), or lobular "neoplasia," is usually discovered when a biopsy is done for some other abnormality. Both breasts are at risk for cancer with this condition. When found, it is generally widely distributed throughout the breast, and frequently bilateral (found in both breasts), though the extent of LCIS found in the breast does not seem to be related to subsequent incidence of breast cancer, according to the National Cancer Institute.(2) NCI states that a patient diagnosed with LCIS has a 25 percent chance of developing an invasive cancer in either breast within 25 years.(2) Infiltrating ductal cancer is the breast cancer that normally develops following LCIS, though invasive lobular carcinoma may also be found.

TREATMENT: Controversial, the options given the patient may be 1) no treatment following biopsy, with careful followup (physical examination plus mammography), or 2) bilateral prophylactic mastectomies (preventive surgical removal of both breasts). Axillary lymph node dissection is not considered necessary with this diagnosis.

NOTE: At times, LCIS, DCIS and atypical hyperplasia are difficult to distinguish in the laboratory. Therefore, a second histopatholic interpretation of the biopsy specimen may be desirable.(2)

Intraductal carcinoma in situ (DCIS) is different from lobular carcinoma in situ (LCIS). It is found in the lining of the breast ducts, rather than the lobules, and is normally found only in one breast, not two. Standard treatment in the past has been the mastectomy.(1) This treatment with added low axillary lymph node dissection results today in a combined and local recurrence rate of one to two percent, though breast conservation treatment is also being used, as well.

Currently, DCIS is detected as microcalcifications or as a soft-tissue abnormality, with several histologic types identified: micropapillary, papillary, solid, cribiform, and comedocarcinoma(possibly more aggressive type).(2) Breast conservation surgery, typically a surgical wide excision with local radiation may be the treatment of choice if a clear margin of safety can be accomplished by surgery. The recurrence rate with this combined treatment is 9-21 percent, with half of these recurrences returning as invasive carcinomas.(2) The incidence of lymph node metastasis is two percent.(1) A mastectomy may be used if recurrence occurs, with a survival rate comparable to mastectomy treatment.(2) Lymph node involvement is rare in DCIS, so dissection is not advocated as standard treatment for this disease.

For the most current information regarding LCIS, DCIS, or atypical hyperplasia, call 1-800-4-Cancer, the National Cancer Institute.

Sources: (1) Interview, Dr. Mukund Sargur, Oncologist, Hematologist, Internist, Evergreen Hospital (Kirkland, WA); (2) "Breast Cancer," *PDQ Information*, #208/00013, 8/01/94.

CAUSES OF BREAST CANCER

The causes for breast cancer are not known. Being a woman and aging seem to be the two highest risk factors for women for breast cancer. There are a number of risk factors that have been identified as increasing the possibility of breast cancer. The following listing is taken primarily from "Overview of Breast Cancer," by Irene Karlsen-Thompson, R.N., M.S.N., O.C.N.(4). "Two-thirds of women diagnosed with breast cancer do not fall in any of known risk categories. Most risks are at such a low level that they only partly explain the high frequency of the disease in the population...Since adult women may not be able to alter their personal risk factors in any practical sense, the best opportunity for reducing mortality is through early detection."(2)

GENETIC FACTORS

Family History

Family history accounts for about five percent of all breast cancers diagnosed. Both maternal and paternal sides are risk factors (breast cancer and prostate cancer.)

- First generation risk is the greatest: mother, sister, daughter ($2\frac{1}{2}$ times).
- Second generation risk: aunt, cousins, grandmothers ($1\frac{1}{2}$ times).
- Higher risk with an increased number of relatives: (e.g., two first-generation relatives equals a four-to-six times higher risk)
- Higher risk with premenopausal and bilateral breast cancers.
- Can skip generations.

CHROMOSOME 17, GENE P53:

If the gene p53 is mutated (altered) in certain ways, it produces the inherited disorder, called Li-Fraumeni Syndrome (LFS). "This syndrome is characterized by an increased susceptibility to breast cancer, soft tissue sarcomas, and several other malignancies, [including] bone cancer, brain tumors, leukemia, and adrenocotical carcinoma), all occurring at unusually early ages."(3) The risk of a number of other cancers may also be elevated, though to a lesser degree. Mutation (alteration) of Gene p53 can occur sporadically (non-familial) during a person's lifetime, as well.(3)

Gene p53 is a tumor suppressor gene, which turns off cell growth. When mutated or damaged, it cannot function properly, which may allow unrestricted cell growth, and, therefore, tumor growth.(3)

One of out of two hundred women may have mutated Gene p53.(3) If mutation is present, she may have a 50 percent chance of developing breast cancer by age 30. Of those who carry the mutated gene, more than 90 percent will develop cancer by age 70.(3)

Call 1-800-4-CANCER (NCI) for latest information on Gene p53.

CHROMOSOME 17, GENE BRCA1:

If the gene BRCA1 is mutated (altered), either by genetic inheritance or sporadically (non-familial), there is a significant increased risk for breast and ovarian cancers. "It is estimated that 45 percent of all families with significantly high breast cancer incidence, and at least 80 percent of families with elevated rates of both early-onset breast cancer and ovarian cancer, carry the mutated BRCA1 gene."(5)

Gene BRCA1 is believed to be a tumor-suppressor gene, which "normally prevent(s) uncontrolled cell proliferation, and its inactivation through loss or mutation can lead to cancer."(5)

One of every two hundred women in the United States may have an inherited mutated Gene BRCA1. If present, there is more than a 50 percent chance of a breast cancer diagnosis by age 50, and 85 percent chance by age 70.(5)

Are Other Genes Implicated in Breast Cancer?

There are many other genes implicated in breast cancer, according to the National Cancer Institute.(5)

Among those presently being studied are:

- BRCA2 mapped to Chromosome 13.
- Ataxia-telangiectasia, linked to the AT gene on Chromosome 11.
- Genes associated with sporadic (non-familial) cases of breast cancer: "…[S]ome have been implicated in causing breast cancer, while others are believed to be involved in later stages of the disease such as invasion and metastasis."(5)
- p53 and AT genes plus a group known as GADD repair genes, a part of "a biochemical pathway…[which together] may be particularly important in the genesis of breast cancer."(5)

Other genes being studied for their roles in breast cancer:

- RB (retinoblastoma) tumor suppressor gene.
- HER-2neu oncogene.
- A number of genes, including the bcl-1 oncogene, involved in the regulation of the cell cycle.
- NM23, metastasis suppressor gene.(5)

Tests Available to the Public for Identifying the Presence of a Genetic Risk (5)

Because so little is fully understood regarding these genes, the tests are at this time only available to those who have cancer, and those considered to have a high family risk. "Of particular concern are discrepancies created between the availability of gene-based diagnostic techniques (such as the anticipated test for BRCA1 mutations) and the lack of effective interventions for the conditions diagnosed…National Cancer Institute (NCI) and the National Center for Human Genome Research (NCHGR) are joining forces in a comprehensive approach to issues around genetic predisposition to cancer."(5)

"Along with NCHGR and NCI, the National Institute for Nursing Research and the National Institute of Mental Health are co-sponsoring a number of pilot projects on counseling for hereditary breast, ovarian, and colon cancer susceptibility. In addition, a task force on genetic testing is being set up in the Department of Health and Human Services to consider these issues, with broad representation from consumers, geneticists and genetic counselors, government officials, and members of the biotechnology community."(5)

ENDOCRINE FACTORS

- *Prolonged Menses:* Women who begin menstruating before 12 years, and late menopause: after 55 years.
- *Exogenous Estrogen:* Taking estrogen supplements may raise risk two to three times if taken over 10 years. High risk for endometrial cancer, also. (Risk decreases when drug is discontinued.) Found to be beneficial in preventing osteoporosis and cardiovascular disease.
- *Birth Control Pills:* Prolonged use before first pregnancy or after age 45 may be risk factors. Risk decreases when drug is discontinued. Protective for uterine and ovarian cancers.
- *Pregnancy:* High risk: no pregnancy, first pregnancy after 30, first pregnancy after 35 (greatest risk). Overall risk two times higher.
- *Miscarriage:* Natural or voluntary, before first full-term pregnancy.

ENVIRONMENTAL FACTORS

- *Western Society:* Affluent, more food available as child.
  - *Fat:* Diet high in fat may be a risk factor.
  - *Obesity:* More of a risk factor for post meno-pausal women
  - *Alcohol:* Increases blood level of estrogen.
  - *Height/Birth Weight:* Some indication of a higher incidence with greater height or birth weight.
- *Pesticides, DDT, PCB:* Four times increase with high blood levels of pesticides.
- *Excessive Radiation Exposure.*

OTHER POSSIBLE FACTORS

- *Large Breast Size:* May "mask" problem (not cause it).
- *Breast Feeding:* May be protective: study results vary.

PROTECTIVE FACTORS

- *Vitamin A:* intake: High vitamin A intake equals decreased breast cancer rate.
- *High (i.e., professional) Level of Athletic Activity:* Possibly protective.

Sources: (1) "Factors That Promote the Development of Human Breast Cancer," by David B. Thomas, *Environmental Health Perspectives*, volume 50, 1983; (2) "Facts and Figures 1993." American Cancer Society; (3) "Family Cancer Syndrome Tied to Gene Defect," *Cancer Facts,* January 1991, pp. 1-4; (4) *Overview of Breast Cancer,* by Irene Karlsen-Thompson, R.N., M.S.N., O.C.N.; (5) "Questions and Answers: The BRCA1 Breast Cancer Susceptibility Gene," *Cancer Facts,* October 4, 1994, pp. 1-7.

Chances of Developing Breast Cancer

By age 25:	… one in 19,608
By age 30:	… one in 2,525
By age 35:	… one in 622
By age 40:	… one in 217
By age 45:	… one in 93
By age 50:	… one in 50
By age 55	… one in 33
By age 60:	… one in 24
By age 65:	… one in 17
By age 70:	… one in 14
By age 75:	… one in 11
By age 80:	… one in 10
By age 85:	… one in 9
Ever:	… one in 8

Y-Me Hotline Newsletter [National Cancer Institute], vol. 38, January/February 1993.

CANCER DETECTION

Breast changes that persist, such as a lump, thickening, swelling, dimpling, skin irritation, distortion, retraction, scaliness, pain, or tenderness of the nipple are the most common warning signs of cancer.(2)

The following chart shows the American Cancer Society's recommended procedures for breast cancer detection:

Procedure	Age	Frequency
BSE (Breast Self Examination)	20 and over	Every month
Breast Physical (Clinical) Exam	20-40	Every 3 years
	Over 40	Every year
Mammography	35-39	Baseline
	40-49	Every 1-2 Years
	50 and over	Every year

REMEMBER.

**Breast Self-Examination
is not a substitute
for routine mammograms or
regular breast exams by a doctor.**

BREAST SELF EXAMINATION (BSE)

This is the way most breast lumps are found. The procedure is simple, free, it can be done on a regular basis, and it is not dangerous. The palpation (feeling an area to detect abnormalities) technique can be simply learned, it is preventive, and it just may save your life. The following is taken from "A Health Guide for All Women," National Cancer Institute #93-3536.

Some research suggests that many women do BSE more thoroughly when they use a pattern of up-and-down lines or strips. Other women feel more comfortable with another pattern. The important thing is to cover the whole breast and to pay special attention to the area between the breast and the underarm, and to the underarm itself. Check the area above the breast, up to the collarbone and all the way over to your shoulder.

LINES: Start in the underarm area and move your fingers downward little by little until they are below the breast. Then move your fingers slightly toward the middle and slowly move back up. Go up and down until you cover the whole area.

CIRCLES: Beginning at the outer edge of your breast, move your fingers slowly around the whole breast in a circle. Move around the breast in smaller and smaller circles, gradually working toward the nipple. Don't forget to check the underarm and upper chest areas, too.

WEDGES: Starting at the outer edge of the breast, move your fingers toward the nipple and back to the edge. Check your whole breast, covering one small wedge-shaped section at a time. Be sure to check the underarm area and the upper chest.

BREAST SELF EXAMINATION STEPS

1) Stand in front of a mirror that is large enough to let you see your breasts clearly. Check both breasts for any thing unusual. Check the skin for puckering, dimpling or scaliness. Look for any discharge from the nipples.

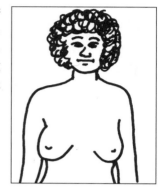

Do steps 2 and 3 to check for any change in the shape or contour of your breasts. As you do these steps, you should feel your chest muscles tighten.

2) Watching closely in the mirror, clasp your hands behind your head and press your hands forward.

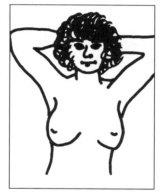

3) Next, press your hands firmly on your hips and bend slightly toward the mirror as you pull your shoulders and elbows forward.

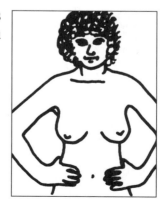

4) Gently squeeze each nipple and look for a discharge.

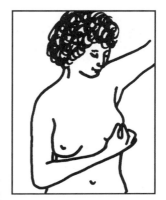

5) Raise one arm. Use the flat part of the fingers of your other hand to check the breast and the surrounding area—firmly, carefully, and thoroughly. Some women like to use lotion or powder to help their fingers glide easily over the skin. Feel for any unusual lump or mass under the skin.

Feel the tissue by pressing your fingers in small, overlapping areas. To be sure you cover your whole breast, take your time and follow a definite pattern: lines, circles, or wedges.

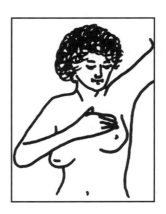

6) It's important to repeat Step 5 while you are lying down. Lie flat on your back, with one arm over your head and a pillow or folded towel under the opposite shoulder. This position flattens the breast and makes it easier to check.

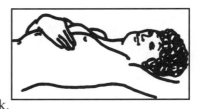

Check each breast and the area around it very carefully, again follow a definite pattern: lines, circles, or wedges.

7) Some women repeat Step 5 in the shower. Your fingers will glide easily over soapy skin, so you can concentrate on feeling for changes underneath.

Call 1-800-ACS-2345 for a free brochure on how to do a Breast Self Examination.

> ***If you notice a lump, a discharge or any other change during the month—whether or not it is during Breast Self Examination—contact your doctor.***

BREAST PHYSICAL (CLINICAL) EXAMINATION

This is done by a physician in the doctor's office. Its particular value is that the exam is done by someone medically educated in palpation techniques used to discover abnormalities.

MAMMOGRAPHY

A mammogram is a low-dose X-ray taken for the purpose of locating the possible presence of a tumor mass in the breast. It is the best available technique by far (over 90% accurate) in detecting small tumors, or microcalcification clusters that may indicate the presence of a tumor mass. Since early detection is the best weapon a woman has against breast cancer, it is a highly recommended screening technique.

Call NCI at 1-800-4-CANCER for more details regarding Mammography Screening.

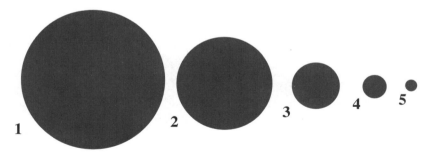

1) Average-sized lump found by women untrained in Breast Self Examination.
2) Average-sized lump found by women practicing occasional Breast Self Examination.
3) Average-sized lump found by women practicing regular Breast Self Examination.
4) Average-sized lump found by first mammogram.
5) Average-sized lump found by regular mammograms.

NOTE: *If a problem is suspected via the use of one of the above techniques, the only way you or your doctor can be sure whether or not it is cancerous is through a biopsy, the specimen of which is then analyzed by a pathologist.*

Sources: (1) *Breast Cancer.* by Yashar Hirshaut, M.D., F.A.C.P. and Peter I. Pressman, M.D., F.A.C.S.; (2) "Cancer Detection: Recommended Health Maintenance Guidelines," American Cancer Society.

DIAGNOSIS OF BREAST CANCER

The diagnosis of breast cancer may be arrived at from many directions. It should be noted that most women discover it for themselves, or seem to have a sense there is something wrong, so go to a doctor to get it checked out, thus getting their suspicions confirmed. Most lumps discovered (over 80 percent) are not cancerous, but rather are fibrous tumors (fibroadenomas), fatty collections, inflammatory masses, infections, or cysts. It is common for benign lesions (noncancerous tumors) in premenopausal patients to enlarge just before menstrual periods, then shrink.(2)

If there is a suspicion of breast cancer, a number of examinations or procedures may be done to check out the possibility more thoroughly.

1) BSE (BREAST SELF EXAMINATION): palpation of the breast done by the patient.

2) CLINICAL EXAMINATION: palpation of the breast done by a qualified physician.

3) MAMMOGRAM: a low-dose X-ray of the breast done in a mammography clinic—the test most respected for its accuracy (over 90 percent accurate) in locating breast cancer.

ALTERNATIVES TO THE MAMMOGRAM:

Breast Ultrasound (Sonography): uses high-frequency sound waves to examine the breast. The pulses of the sound waves created by the interaction with the breast tissue and/or tumor are recorded on a screen, then photographed. It cannot locate micro-calcifications or very small tumors, so is not recommended as screening tool. It can be useful as a follow up to mammogram to record density; a cyst is liquid filled, so the sound wave will go right through it, as opposed to a solid lump (fibroadenoma) or a cancer, which will make the sound waves bounce right back, creating a different pattern.

Thermography: a special camera measures and records the heat pattern of the breast. Not found to be very effective in locating breast cancers, though experimented with for over 30 years.(1)

Transillumination (diaphanography): the breast is lit up with infrared radiation (transilluminated), with the observation that cancerous tissue absorbs more infrared than normal tissue. No reliable evidence that it is as good as mammography in screening for breast cancer.

CAT Scan (Computerized Axial Tomography): "uses radiation to create cross-sectional pictures that are combined to create extremely detailed images."(1) This procedure is expensive, uses more radiation than mammography, and requires use of intravenous contrast material that may entail some risks.(1) It is valuable for identification of density of material, but not normally used in screening for breast cancer.

MRI (Magnetic Resonance Imaging): image created by using a magnetic field, rather than radiation. Expensive, presently experimental in viewing the breast.

Xeromammography: Developed by Xerox, this is a form of mammographic exam that creates a blue image on white paper. It is used by some physicians, but is not as accurate as mammography. The machine is no longer being manufactured.(1)

4) BIOPSY:

Fine Needle Aspiration: used to determine if a lesion is cystic or solid.(2) If liquid can be drained from the lesion, no blood is removed, no abnormal cells are found, and if the lesion does not return within two weeks, it is diagnosed as a cyst, and treatment is ended.(2) About five percent of aspirations done do not detect cancer when it is present.

Stereotactic Fine Needle Biopsy: computer-assisted X-rays guide a needle to the precise position of a lesion, or localized microcalcification, which then extracts some of the lesion for analysis by a pathologist.

Incisional Biopsy: the surgical removal of a small piece of a tumor to determine whether or not it is cancer. This is done on an outpatient basis or in the doctor's office.

Excisional Biopsy: the surgical removal of a small tumor to determine whether or not it is cancer. This is done on an outpatient basis or in the doctor's office.

One-Stage Procedure: A woman goes in for a biopsy and comes out with a mastectomy (loss of her breast) completed. This is seldom done today because of the pressure from women to stop it, since significant decisions were being made with regard to her body, without her input while she was asleep on the operating table. There are times when it this is appropriate, but it needs to be a joint decision between the surgeon and patient before surgery.

Two-Stage Procedure: The biopsy is performed first, and at a later date, days or weeks later, after the patient has had time to fully examine the options open to her/him, the second surgical procedure (lumpectomy, mastectomy, etc.) is performed. This is the most common procedure used today.

---

5) ADDITIONAL TESTS may be done, if cancer is confirmed, to determine whether cancer is located elsewhere in the body:

X-ray of the chest (or other areas): to assess if cancer is located in lungs or ribs.

Bone Scan: to check for cancer spread to the bone.

Abdominal CT (CAT Scan): to check for liver involvement, especially if the serum alkaline phosphatase (a bone and liver enzyme) is elevated.(2)

Sources: (1) *Breast Cancer,* Yashar Hirshaut, M.D., F.A.C.P. and Peter I. Pressman, M.D., F.A.C.S.; (2) *Everyone's Guide to Cancer Therapy,* by Malin Dollinger, M.D., Ernest H. Rosenbaum, M.D., and Greg Cable; (3) *Overview of Breast Cancer,* Irene Karlsen-Thompson, R.N., M.S.N., O.C.N.

NEW TECHNIQUES BEING STUDIED

1) *Nuclear medicine imaging PET scan*, with the radioactive isotope FDG, has been studied for breast cancer detection, but is not being considered for screening at this time. The procedure is still considered experimental. Also, it is very expensive, at $1,500 per test compared to less than $100 for mammography.(2)

2) *Nipple aspirate cytology* has been shown to detect early breast cancer in women 35-50, who are neither pregnant nor lactating. It is being considered as an early screening technique.

TECHNIQUE: A "Sartorius breast pump," consisting of a suction cup attached by a short plastic tube to a 10 cc syringe is placed over the nipple. Negative pressure (for about 15 seconds) is created by withdrawing the plunger in the syringe to 6 or 7 ccs. When successful, a drop or more of liquid is obtained, which then can be studied for abnormalities.

It is suggested that this procedure could be "readily incorporated into a routine physical examination along with breast palpation. There is no evidence of risk to the patient." Additional diagnostic modalities such as mammogram and biopsy are needed to complete the clinical diagnosis when atypical (abnormal) cells are found.(3)

Sources: (1) Interview, Dr. Mukund Sargur, Oncologist, Hematologist, Internist, Evergreen Hospital, (Kirkland, WA); (2) "New Technologies Proving Useful for Breast Cancer Diagnosis, *Journal of the National Cancer Institute* 85(2):88-90, January 20, 1993; (3) "Nipple Aspirate Cytology in High-Risk BCa Identification," by Margaret Wrensch, Ph.D., and Nicholas Petrakis, M.D., *Contemporary Oncology* November 1994, pp. 37-45.

PROGNOSTIC FACTORS

"Cancer survival statistics are averages based on large numbers of patients. They cannot be used to predict what will happen to one person. A patient's prospects for recovery (prognosis) can be affected by many factors, including the type of cancer and whether it has spread; the patient's age, general health, and response to treatment; and other variables. Only the doctor who is familiar with a patient's case knows enough about that person to discuss the prognosis. It is important to understand, however, that even the doctor who is familiar with the patient's medical history and current condition cannot tell the patient exactly what to expect."

— "Statistics/Prognosis," *Cancer Facts,* 2/26/93

The following section is taken largely from *Overview of Breast Cancer,* by Irene Karlsen-Thompson, R.N., M.S.N., O.C.N.:

1) THE PRESENCE OR ABSENCE OF CANCER IN THE LYMPH NODES under the arm (axillary nodes) on the affected side. If present, the number of lymph nodes involved, plus the pattern of involvement becomes significant in treatment choices. Can also be found in cervical, supraclavicular, and intraclavicular lymph nodes on the chest and neck area. The presence or absence of lymph nodes is the single most important factor in treatment choice.(1) (0 nodes, most favorable; 1-3 nodes also includes lymphatic vessel invasion; over 4 nodes, less favorable; over 10 nodes, least favorable).(3)

2) PREMENOPAUSAL/POSTMENOPAUSAL STATUS, plus AGE OF PATIENT. Treatment choices differ significantly depending on these three factors.

3) POSITIVE OR NEGATIVE ESTROGEN/PROGESTERONE RECEPTOR STATUS, which indicates whether or not there are proteins present in the breast that are able (positive) or unable (negative) to bind estrogen or progesterone, which then can be substituted by hormones (e.g., Tamoxifen [Nolvadex]), an

estrogen-blocker) in treatment to discourage the growth of cancer cells. Mature (Well-differentiated) cells are those that typically produced large numbers of estrogen and progesterone receptors, as opposed to immature (Poorly Differentiated, Undifferentiated) cells. Mature cells also indicate to the pathologist that the cells have taken time to grow and develop, which means the cancer is probably more slow-growing.(4)

4) SIZE OF TUMOR: The larger tumors may be associated with a higher rate of recurrence within the breast, in the local area, or at a distant site.(2)

5) METASTASIS: The degree of breast cancer spread via the blood or lymphatic system to other sites in the body (e.g., bone, liver, brain, lungs).

6) PATHOLOGY OF TUMOR: The appearance of the cancer cells under a microscope, or by other techniques in a laboratory, performed by a pathologist.

Aneuploid versus Diploid: The use of flow cytometry determines whether an abnormal (aneuploid) or normal (diploid) number of chromosomes is present in the DNA material of the cell. When the cells have lost their ability to fully control chromosome duplication(2) in a normal way, it is considered a poorer prognosis.

Nuclear Grade: How much the nucleus of the cancer cell looks like the nucleus of a normal cell (G1-G3: G1 the best).

S Phase: Flow cytometry is one of the tests used to determine how many cells at a given time are in the S phase (synthesizing DNA in preparation for dividing) at the time of the test.(2) Seven percent of cells in this phase is commonly considered unfavorable by pathologists.

Cell Proliferation: the rate of the cells multiplying is an indication of the aggressiveness of the cancer cells.

Presence and Heightened Activity of Oncogenes: When certain genes, such as HER-2neu (erb-2), EGFR, or C-myc are in high number, this is associated with the potential for more aggressive cancer growth.

Cathepsin D: The production of this enzyme is controlled by estrogen. High levels of Cathepsin D present in node-negative tumors (normally a good prognosis) is an indicator of a poor prognosis.(2)

Gene p53 (located on Chromosome 17): If mutation of this gene (a change from its normal structure) is present, it may indicate a more aggressive cancer.

Gene BRCA1 (located on Chromosome 17): If mutation of this gene (a change from its normal structure) is present, it may indicate a more aggressive cancer.

Tumor Angiogenesis: The number of micro-blood vessels in the tumor indicates a greater probability of recurrence, particularly with Stage 1 and 2, node-negative.

NOTE: *Any one of these factors alone (including others presently being explored) does not give a full picture for the oncologist. All available factors at the time of diagnosis must be put together in a complex picture to construct the very best individual treatment plan for the patient.*

TO THE PATIENT:

It is essential that you choose a board-certified oncologist to oversee your treatment plan, one who is experienced, competent, and respectful of your individual needs and concerns. Anti-cancer drugs are highly toxic and must be administered with great care and respect for the individual patient. The breast cancer surgeon is usually the best person to recommend a qualified oncologist. However, if you are not satisfied, you can call the American Cancer Society 1-800-ACS-2345 for information regarding qualified oncologists in your area.

Sources: (1) "Adjuvant Therapy for Breast Cancer," American Cancer Society #5555, 1993; (2) *Breast Cancer,* by Dr. Yashar Hirshaut, M.D., F.A.C.P. and Peter I. Pressman, M.D., F.A.C.S.; (3) *Overview of Breast Cancer,* by Irene Karlsen-Thompson, R.N, M.S.N, O.C.N; (4) Mukund Sargur, M.D., Oncologist, Hematologist, Internist.

STAGING OF BREAST CANCER

Staging was developed by the American Joint Committee on Cancer and International Union Against Cancer in an attempt to categorize the different stages of various cancers around the world so that a standardized treatment plan could be approached by the international medical community.

Staging of breast cancer is based on three factors: 1) Tumor size (T), 2) Node involvement (N), and 3) Metastasis (Spread of the cancer). The three factors are abbreviated by the acronym "TNM."

BREAST CANCER STAGES

Stage 0:   In situ carcinoma, intraductal or lobular carcinoma, or Paget's disease of the nipple with no tumor.

Stage I: A tumor no larger than 2 centimeters (about 1 inch) that has not spread outside the breast.

Stage II: A tumor no larger than 2 centimeters that has spread to the lymph nodes under the arm (the axillary lymph nodes) OR

a tumor between 2 and 5 centimeters (from 1 to 2 inches) and may or may not have spread to the lymph nodes under the arm OR

a tumor larger than 5 centimeters (larger than 2 inches) and has no or minimal spread to the lymph nodes under the arm.

Stage IIIA: A tumor that is smaller than 5 centimeters and has spread to the lymph nodes under the arm, which have grown into each other or into other structures and are attached to them OR

a tumor that is bigger than 5 centimeters and has spread to the lymph nodes under the arm.

Stage IIIB: A tumor that has spread to tissue near the breast (chest wall, including the ribs and the muscles to the chest) OR

a tumor that has spread to lymph nodes near the collarbone.

Stage IV: A tumor that has spread to other organs of the body, most often the bones, lungs, liver, or brain.

NOTE: *The above consolidations of each stage are the most easily accessible I have found for quick lay reference, taken mainly from "Breast Cancer," PDQ Information for Patients, National Cancer Institute, 10/31/94. For more detailed information on TNM staging, call the National Cancer Institute, 1-800-4-CANCER.*

FIVE-YEAR SURVIVAL RATES

BREAST CANCER STAGES AND FIVE-YEAR SURVIVAL RATES

Stage 0 ....95% Survival Rate

Stage 1 ....85% Survival Rate

Stage 2 ....66% Survival Rate

Stage 3 ....41% Survival Rate

Stage 4 ....10% Survival Rate

"Breast Cancer," National Cancer Institute #208/00013, 8/1/94

It is *essential* to understand that these rates are simply a measure used to determine how many women in a particular stage of breast cancer were alive to be counted at the end of a five-year period, i.e., "a measure scientists use to compare the value of one treatment with another."(5) The rates are *not* predictable of an individual's personal outcome. *In every stage, even the most advanced, there are survivors who may live to a ripe old age.*

The American Cancer Society's *1994 Estimated Cancer Incidence by Site and Sex* indicates that it is estimated that breast cancer for women will have the highest incidence of diagnosis of any cancers this year (32 percent), with lung cancer coming in second (13 percent). However, the estimated mortalities for women's cancers this year indicate the highest rate in lung cancer (23 percent), and the second highest rate in breast cancer (18 percent).

FIVE-YEAR SURVIVAL RATES

Localized breast cancer: 93%

Breast Cancer in situ (non-invasive): approaches 100%

Breast Cancer spread regionally: 71%

Breast Cancer with distant metastasis: 18%

"Facts and Figures 1993," American Cancer Society.

Sources: (1) *Breast Cancer,* by Yashar Hirshaut, M.D., F.A.C.P., and Peter I. Pressman, M.D., F.A.C.S.; (2) *Everyone's Guide to Cancer Therapy,* by Malin Dollinger, M.D., Ernest H. Rosenbaum, M.D., and Greg Cable; (3) *The Breast Cancer Companion,* by Kathy LaTour; (4) "Adjuvant Therapy for Breast Cancer," American Cancer Society #5555, 1993; (5) *Cancer Facts,* National Cancer Institute, 2/26/93.

BREAST CANCER IN PREGNANT WOMEN
(Excerpt from an interview with Dr. Mukund Sargur)

C: How do you treat pregnant women who develop breast cancer?

S: This is a difficult problem. Most pregnant women who develop breast cancer have a delay in diagnosis. The swelling of the breast during pregnancy can easily hide a breast lump, and since mammograms are not done during pregnancy (due to the possible risk of fetal exposure to radiation), its detection is usually delayed.

Because breast cancer during pregnancy occurs rarely—one to three percent of all breast cancer cases; or, 3 out of every 10,000 pregnancies(3), both the doctor and the patient may not consider or explore the possibility as seriously, thus contributing to a delayed diagnosis.

1st TRIMESTER: When detected in this phase of pregnancy, therapeutic abortion is considered. If the cancer is very small, a lumpectomy (or other conservation surgical types), or mastectomy, without chemotherapy and radiation are options.(3)

2nd or 3rd TRIMESTER: If detected in either of these phases of pregnancy, both a lumpectomy and a mastectomy are options; chemotherapy is an option for advanced breast cancer. Adriamycin (doxorubicin) and vincristine can be given in second and third trimester. 5-FU (fluorouracil) and methotrexate are not recommended. Radiation therapy is not recommended.

"Breast cancer during pregnancy is one of the most difficult management problems. The diagnosis usually involves a host of psychosocial, ethical, religious, legal, and medical considerations, all requiring multidisciplinary consultations and intense psychological support. Both staging and treatment are complicated by pregnancy...The patient, her family, clergy, and the medical team have to work closely together to balance ethical, moral, religious, and medical concerns in order to provide the best outcome for the woman (and the baby, if possible)."(3)

CONCLUSION: *Be aware that breast cancer can occur during a pregnancy, so be aggressive in pursuing anything suspicious in the breast with your doctor. Early diagnosis offers the best options for treatment and cure. "With appropriate use of surgery, combination chemotherapy and radiotherapy, the main therapeutic options for women with breast cancer can be offered and prognosis equivalent to that occurring in the nonpregnant patient can be achieved."(3)*

Sources: (1) Interview, Dr. Mukund Sargur, Oncologist, Hematologist, Internist, Evergreen Hospital (Kirkland, WA); (2) *The Breast Cancer Companion*, by Kathy LaTour; (3)"Management of Breast Cancer in the Pregnant Patient," by Stephen E. Jones, M.D., *Contemporary Oncology.* 2(6): 19-24, July/August 1992.

TYPES OF MASTECTOMY

PARTIAL OR SEGMENTAL MASTECTOMY

*Includes Quadrantectomy, which is the removal of
about one-quarter of the breast tissue—less commonly used.*

The partial or segmental mastectomy is a surgical procedure in which the tumor plus a section of normal tissue surrounding it, including some skin and the the lining of the chest muscle below the tumor, are removed. In some cases, some or all of the lymph nodes under the arm (axillary nodes) are removed also to check for possible cancer spread.

Advantages: In a large breast, the breast shape is mostly reserved, with little possibility of the loss of muscle strength or swelling in the arm (lymphedema).

Disadvantages: In a small- or medium-sized breast, the breast shape is noticeably altered, with some possibility of swelling in the arm (lymphedema).

LUMPECTOMY

The lumpectomy surgical procedure in which only the breast lump is removed, plus a margin of normal tissue surrounding it (for safety), usually followed by radiation therapy, (*see* Radiation Therapy) and the removal of some of the underarm lymph nodes (axillary nodes) to test for possible cancer spread.

Advantages: The breast is not removed.

Disadvantages: Small-breasted women with large lumps usually have a noticeably altered breast shape, with some possibility of swelling in the arm (lymphedema). Scar tissue may make breast cancer detection more difficult in the future.

MODIFIED RADICAL MASTECTOMY

Total Mastectomy with Axillary (Underarm) Dissection

The modified radical mastectomy is surgical procedure in which the breast, the underarm lymph nodes (axillary nodes), and the lining over the chest muscles are removed. Occasionally the smaller of the two chest muscles (pectoralis minor) is also removed. Currently this is the most common treatment of early stage breast cancer.

Advantages: The chest muscle and muscle strength of the arm are preserved. Arm swelling (lymphedema) is less likely, or milder than that observed in a radical mastectomy. Cosmetic appearance is better, and reconstruction easier than in a radical. Survival is equal to radical mastectomy when treated in early stages.

Disadvantages: Removal of breast. May be arm swelling (lymphedema) due to lymph node removal.

TOTAL OR SIMPLE MASTECTOMY

The total or simple mastectomy is a surgical procedure in which only the breast is removed, and sometimes a few of the underarm lymph nodes (axillary nodes) to check for cancer spread. Radiation therapy may follow.

Advantages: Chest muscles are left intact, as well as arm strength. Most, perhaps all, of underarm lymph nodes (axillary nodes) are left, so the risk of arm swelling (lymphedema) is reduced. Breast reconstruction is easier than modified radical mastectomy.

Disadvantages: Breast removal. If cancer spread has occurred to lymph nodes under the arm (axillary nodes), it may go undiscovered.

TOTAL GLANDULAR MASTECTOMY

The total glandular mastectomy is a surgical procedure in which all of the breast tissue is removed, leaving just the skin available for reconstruction. The nipple and areola are also typically removed, to be replaced in reconstruction.

Advantages: All breast tissue, thus all microscopic possibilities of breast cancer cells in the breast itself, is removed, with only the patient's skin still intact. If successful, good possible cosmetic effect.

Disadvantages: A significant risk for skin necrosis, or skin death, due to the fact that not enough tissue is available—just the skin—for available blood flow. Not a promise of cure, since breast cancer is systemic, and may have already metastasized to another location via the blood or lymphatic system.

RADICAL MASTECTOMY (HALSTED'S)

The radical mastectomy is a surgical procedure in which the entire breast, axillary lymph nodes and all chest muscles are removed. This procedure is seldom used today due to the large degree of disfigurement of the woman's body due to the extensive surgery, with no curative advantage to the patient when compared to other current breast cancer treatments available.

Advantages: Seldom considered advantageous today. Using the radical mastectomy as a standard treatment was supported in the past by the medical belief that breast cancer was a local disease. The theory was that the more potentially contaminated tissue the surgeon could remove, the greater the chance for patient survival. With present knowledge, it is understood that breast cancer is a systemic disease which can multiply uncontrollably, and travel via the blood and lymphatic system to other locations in the body. Therefore, the justification for the extensive disfigurement of the woman's body in a radical mastectomy is seldom present. (*See* Dr. Mukund Sargur's Interview for further information.)

Disadvantages: Extensive disfigurement, high risk of lymphedema due to extensive removal of lymph nodes, muscle weakness in shoulder and arm due to extensive chest muscle removal. Seldom used, since there is a question of any curative advantage in the use of this treatment when compared with what is presently available with the combined treatments of surgery, chemotherapy, radiation, and hormone treatment.

PROPHYLACTIC MASTECTOMY

A prophylactic mastectomy is the surgical removal of a breast, or both breasts to reduce the risk of cancer due to the possibility of high risk for breast cancer, but without a confirmed diagnosis. This is a choice made by some women with a high family risk, a history of chronic benign breast problems with or without several biopsies, mammograms that show findings more and more difficult to interpret, or a history of breast cancer in the other breast. The surgery may involve a total mastectomy (removal of the whole breast), or just the breast tissue (subcutaneous mastectomy), leaving the skin and the nipple intact.

There is controversy over whether or not it is a wise choice for a woman.

The American Cancer Society states the following: "The American Cancer Society approves the concept of reconstruction, when appropriate, for women who have had a mastectomy. However, the Society has great concern about prophylactic mastectomies. Only very strong clinical and/or pathological indications warrant doing this type of 'preventive' operation."(1)

If a woman is considering a prophylactic mastectomy, it is important that she discuss thoroughly with her doctor "the procedure, reconstructive surgery, potential complications, and follow-up care."(1)

Some insurances question coverage of this procedure. The patient may or may not choose a course of reconstructive surgery: It is a personal choice.

Advantages: The removal of the possibility of future development of breast cancer due to the removal of the breast tissue. Peace of mind.

Disadvantages: The total removal of both breasts, a difficult choice for most women. Possibility that the breast or breasts removed may never have developed breast cancer. Psychological adjustment.

NOTE: *There is no consistent evidence that timing of a mastectomy with regard to the menstrual cycle has an impact on either overall or disease-free survival.(3)*

Sources: (1) "Prophylactic Mastectomy," American Cancer Society #5620, 1993; (2) *Breast Cancer,* by Yashar Hirshaut, M.D., F.A.C.P. and Peter I. Pressman, M.D., F.A.C.S.; (3) "Breast Cancer," National Cancer Institute, *PDQ Information* #208/00013.

LYMPH NODE REMOVAL

Lymph node removal is the surgical removal of some or all of the regional lymph nodes which are then dissected in the laboratory to determine if cancer cells are present. If "positive" (present), it tells the doctor that the patient's breast cancer may have spread and is growing elsewhere (metastasized) in the body. The number of lymph nodes in which cancer is found, (involved with cancer, lymph node involvement) is significant in "staging" the patient's breast cancer, which determines the course of medical treatment recommended.

The lymph nodes "act as our first line of defense against infections and cancer."(2) They are small oval-shaped organs "connected by small vessels called lymphatics" that produce lymphocytes. Lymphocytes fight infection in the body, and "also filter out and destroy bacteria, foreign substances and cancer cells."(2)

Sources: (1) "Breast Cancer: Understanding Treatment Options," National Cancer Institute #87-2675; (2) *Everyone's Guide to Cancer Therapy,* by Malin Dollinger, M.D., Ernest H. Rosenbaum, M.D., and Greg Cable; (3) "Mastectomy: A Treatment for Breast Cancer," National Cancer Institute #87-658.

Lymphedema

Lymphedema, or swelling of the arm, was more common when radical mastectomies were performed, followed by radiation treatment. The procedures interfered with lymph drainage in the arm, which then caused swelling. When the lymph nodes are removed with a modified radical mastectomy, about 5% of women develop lymphedema. Fewer problems are seen with women who have lumpectomies.

However, it is important for women to be aware of the symptoms of lymphedema, so that immediate attention can be given to them when they begin, rather than waiting until they become a more serious condition.

"Lymphedema usually begins with swelling in the hands..."(2) If there is persistent swelling in the hand and/or arm following surgery, seek medical advice. Early diagnosis and treatment are important for the best curative result. Untreated, lymphedema can cause increased swelling, with accompanying complications, and infection of the swollen area, with even more serious results.(2)

To prevent symptoms following surgery, the following is recommended:

- Wear gloves while doing housework or gardening to prevent infections.
- *Never* allow an injection or blood drawing on the side of the body where the lymph nodes were taken out.
- *Never* have blood pressures taken in the arm where the lymph nodes were taken out.
- Do not wear tight jewelry or elastic bands around affected fingers or arms.
- Avoid cutting cuticles when manicuring hands.
- Elevate arm whenever possible to assist lymphatic flow.
- Exercise arm regularly in moderation to keep it healthy, as you would any other part of the body.

Call the National Lymphedema Network at 1-800-541-3259 for more information.

Sources: (1) *Breast Cancer,* by Dr. Yashar Hirshaut, M.D., F.A.C.P. and Dr. Peter I. Pressman, M.D., F.A.C.S.; (2) *Lymphedema, An Information Booklet,* 3rd ed, rev., by Saskia R.J. Thiadens, R.N., National Lymphedema Network.

ARM EXERCISES FOLLOWING SURGERY

A series of exercises are recommended following surgery to regain the full rotation of the arm, and to assist the re-establishment of the lymphatic system which was interrupted due to the removal of a number of the lymph nodes during surgery. The doctor may recommend exercises for the patient to do. A Reach for Recovery volunteer is usually available to visit the patient in the hospital, who demonstrates the recommended exercises to the patient before she/he returns home. If not, a volunteer can be contacted by the American Cancer Society, 1-800-ACS-2345.

BREAST PROSTHESES

The first prosthesis a woman will have who has just had a mastectomy may come from a volunteer from Reach to Recovery, (from the American Cancer Society), a day or so after the mastectomy surgery in the hospital. This prosthesis will be a soft, fiber-filled form designed to fit in her bra.

When it is time to look for a more permanent prosthesis, be aware that there are many sizes, shapes (plus several shades of color), and costs to choose from. There are different shapes and sizes of free-form prostheses, usually filled with a liquid, or semi-liquid solution or gel, such as silicone, approaching the feel of a real breast. There is a new type available that can adhere to the skin with a strip of adhesive material. The average cost of most available prostheses runs between $150 and $250 each, without the bra. At least part of the cost is usually covered by insurance, but it is advisable to check with your insurance company before purchase, or call National Insurance Consumer Helpline, 1-800-942-4242. If it is not covered, call the American Cancer Society, which helps women who need a prosthesis, but who do not have the funds available to purchase one.

It is important to have a permanent prosthesis that is *weighted,* so that there is not an adverse effect on balance and posture.

SUGGESTION: *After about a year and a half of using a silicone filled prosthesis, breast cancer survivor Marie Baker showed me her washable, weighted prosthesis, built into an "active bra," available through the Sears Shop At Home service for less than most others. (It was about $70 each for the bra with built-in prosthesis about six years ago (one side); now they run about $100 each, plus tax). Designed by a breast cancer survivor, it is a great value.*

The prosthesis, "Nearly Me, Rest Breast," available through Nordstrom's and other shops, I have found to be the best-made, all-around form to use for lingerie, swim suits, and occasionally for insertion in other bras. They run about $50 each. (I swim five days a week in chlorine water: these forms have lasted over two years each, which is twice as long as any others I have used).

A complete list of available prostheses in your area is available by calling the American Cancer Society, or get in touch with Reach to Recovery, 1-800-ACS-2345.

BREAST RECONSTRUCTION

Breast reconstruction is the surgical recreation of a breast mound, instead of using a prosthesis (an artificial breast form placed inside a brassiere). Breast reconstruction can be done by the use of implants, or by the use of the patient's own tissues. The procedure is not always covered by insurance, so if this is a factor, call your insurance company to find out for sure.

A board-certified plastic surgeon who is experienced in breast reconstruction is the doctor most qualified to perform such a surgery. The commitment of about a year or so of a patient's time and energies needs to be made available to complete the procedures required for a breast reconstruction. Some women have reconstruction done immediately following a mastectomy (immediate reconstruction); others wait several months or even years (delayed reconstruction).

When breast contour following modified radical mastectomy is to be restored using a tissue flap, the need for blood transfusions should be anticipated. *"It is strongly recommended that the patient make arrangements to donate his/her own blood for surgery to assure its quality."* ("Breast Cancer," *PDQ Information,* 12/5/94)

It normally takes two-to-three surgeries for a complete breast reconstruction, depending on:

1) whether the initial surgery is done immediately following a mastectomy in the hospital,

2) the choices made for reconstruction,

3) the professional qualifications, experience, skill and judgment of the surgeon,

4) the tolerance of the body to the necessary procedures, and the ability of the body to respond with the appropriate healing, and

5) the commitment and/or ability of the patient to support full recovery.

PATIENT'S OPTIONS

1) the replacement of the breast mound (newly reconstructed breast without the nipple),

2) the replacement of areola,

3) the replacement of the nipple, and sometimes,

4) surgical altering of the remaining breast to more closely match to newly constructed breast. When all goes well, the end product can be quite remarkable. However, the patient needs to be aware that, as in all surgery, there are risks involved, and that the end result might not always be the one hoped for, depending on what happens along the way.

If a patient is considering breast reconstruction, these are things to keep in mind:

1) *Interview two or three plastic surgeons before making a final decision.* You will be amazed at the differences, and will be able to sort out those who would not be a fit for you. (You wouldn't think of choosing a dress or suit without trying on several to see which one you really like. How much more important to choose carefully the doctor who may surgically alter your body forever.)

2) *Insist on a plastic surgeon who is board-certified.* (There are, unfortunately, doctors who advertise in the yellow pages as plastic surgeons who are not qualified to do so, the end results of which can be devastating to the patient and loved ones. (Call 1-800-ACS-2345 for a listing of qualified plastic surgeons in your area.)

3) *Choose a plastic surgeon who is experienced with breast reconstructions for the best result,* and knowledge of possible complications. Ask the doctor how many he/she has performed, for pictures, and personal contacts with patients willing to share with you how it is to go through the procedure.

4) *Choose a plastic surgeon who respects you and your concerns.* It is your life and your body, after all. Never forget it. You should

have final say in every decision along the way, and be respected for it, or consider finding another plastic surgeon.

NOTE: Augmentation *is when an implant is surgically inserted to increase the size of the breast appearance. Not considered breast reconstruction, since the original breast mound is still intact.*

BREAST MOUND RECONSTRUCTION OPTIONS

The surgical options which may be available to the patient for breast mound reconstruction are: 1) an *Expander* and/or the *Surgical Insertion of an Implant,* or 2) a *Flap Technique* using the patient's own tissue to reconstruct a breast mound. Both surgical options offer to the patient the possibility of areola and nipple reconstruction, which are done in separate surgical procedures. The patient may, depending on treatments necessary, have an *immediate reconstruction* (at the time of the mastectomy), or a *post-mastectomy reconstruction*, which may follow a mastectomy by several months, or even years.

POSSIBLE COMPLICATIONS

Capsular Contracture: This is a common complication of implantations throughout the body. The body reacts to the foreign body, in this case the breast implant, by forming a "hard scar tissue sack" (fibrous tissue) around its surface, resulting in hardened, sometimes painful areas in the breast.(1,5) It can be corrected by surgical removal or breaking up of the hardened scar tissue, and replant replacement. Some women have repeated problems with this; others, no problem at all. New implants are covered with a textured surface which reduces the probability of the formation of scar tissue.

Skin Necrosis: "Skin Death," a complication that can occur following any type of reconstructive surgery due to an interrupted, and eventually, inadequate blood supply.

NOTE: *An optimum surgical result is greatly complicated if the patient smokes, since the microscopic blood flow to the skin, as well as other areas of the body (such as bones) can be greatly impaired by smoking. Some plastic surgeons refuse to do plastic surgery on a patient who smokes, since the healing process is impeded by the lack of normal blood flow; this significantly increases the risk of complications. The surgeon may request that a patient stop smoking for a period of time before surgery.(5)*

OPTIONS

Implants

Approximately 2 million women in the United States have had breast implants over the past 20 to 30 years, most for cosmetic "augmentative" (enlargement) purposes;(4) but implants are used increasingly by women with breast cancer as an option.

There are *Nonflap* and *Flap* procedures available in breast reconstruction. A patient needs to be fully informed of the choices available to her, given her unique circumstances.

Nonflap Procedures

Simple Versus Tissue Expansion

The Simple Nonflap Procedure involves the use of existing tissue, including muscle, at the mastectomy site. Using the mastectomy scar for incision when possible, the implant is simply inserted under the muscle.

Nonflap Procedure with Tissue Expansion involves the use of "a temporary internal breast implant called a tissue expander," which is placed in the position where a permanent implant will be located. A saline solution is injected into the implant over a

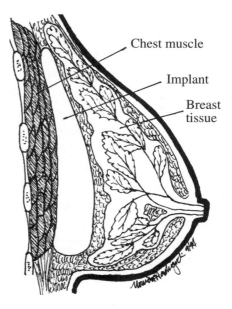

Chest muscle

Implant

Breast tissue

period of weeks, a small amount at a time, which stretches the breast skin to the desired size. This can cause the patient some discomfort. At this point, the expansion implant is removed, and the permanent implant is inserted into position.(3)

Silicone Implant

This is a silicone rubber envelope filled with soft, silicone gel that feels like very thick jelly. The envelope may have either a smooth or textured surface.

Medical concerns regarding the safety of silicone implants for women prompted the Food and Drug Administration in January 1992 to call for "a moratorium on the use of silicone gel breast implants until new information on their safety can be thoroughly reviewed by an independent advisory panel and the agency can make a final decision in light of the panel's review."(2)

Patient Value: The replacement of the natural breast which has been surgically removed, with a natural looking breast shape.

Side Effects (Known): Capsular contracture, which is a hardening of the scar tissue that normally forms around the implant. "This can...cause pain, hardening of the breast or changes in its appearance.(1)

Calcium deposits, can form in the surrounding tissue, which can cause pain and harding of the breast.

Possible rupture, allowing the gel filling to be released into the surrounding tissue. Possible removal of the implant, if severe problems result.

Temporary or permanent changes in nipple or breast sensation can result, due to the surgery.

Side Effects (Possible): The tiny amounts of silicone, or "sweat" ("gel bleed") through the lining of an intact implant has been suggested to be connected to certain auto-immune (connective tissue) diseases such as lupus, scleroderma, and rheumatoid arthritis in some women. Conclusive data is not yet in, so cautionary measures are in place. The silicone implants are only available to breast cancer patients, or for replacement of silicone implants already in place, not for cosmetic surgery.

Possible obstruction or increased difficulty of identifying cancer either by palpation or mammography, according to the American Cancer Society.

Contact the FDA (Food and Drug Administration) at 1-301-443-5006 for the most current information regarding silicone implants.

Saline-Filled Implant

This is a silicone rubber envelope filled during surgery with sterile salt water (saline solution). Currently this is the most common implant used for reconstruction.

Advantages: the creation of a breast shape to replace the natural breast removed during surgery.

Side Effects (Known): Capsular contracture (hardening of the scar tissue surrounding the implant), with accompanying pain, hardening of the breast, and appearance changes in the breast.

Calcium deposit formation around the implant area, with the same possible symptoms as seen in capsular contracture.

Rupture more likely with saline-filled implant, so care should be taken "to avoid trauma to the breast such as might occur from falls or very active sports."(1) If rupture does occur, it typically deflates rapidly, flagging the problem, so that it can be surgically replaced.

Some obstruction and increased difficulty in being able to locate the presence of breast cancer either by palpation or mammography. Recommend patient go to a mammography center where the medical personnel is experienced in doing mammography for implant patients. Additional X-ray pictures need to be taken (three-to-four, instead of two) to view the breast accurately, which will add some cost to the procedure.

Double Lumen Implant

This implant has two silicone rubber envelopes, one inside the other. One is filled with silicone gel by the manufacturer. The other is filled during surgery with a small amount of saline solution. This permits the surgeon to adjust the size. This is less commonly used.

Call 1-800-635-0635 (24-hour referral service number) to obtain names of board-certified plastic surgeons in your area who are active members of the American Society of Plastic and Reconstructive Surgeons, Inc.

Sources: (1) *FDA Backgrounder: Current and Useful Information from the Food and Drug Administration,* August 1991; (2) *Silicone Gel Implants,* CIS bulletin from the Fred Hutchinson Cancer Research Center, January 1992; (3) "Breast Reconstruction," American Cancer Society #5071; (4) "Silicone Gel Breast Implants," American Cancer Society #2666; (5) O*verview of Silicone Gel-Filled Breast Implants,* by the American Society of Plastic and Reconstructive Surgeons, June 1992.

Flap Reconstruction

Lats Flap (Latissimus Dorsi Flap Reconstruction)

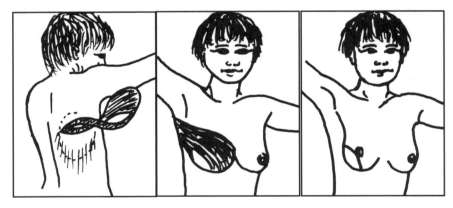

| Latissimus dorsi muscle and skin flap raised. | Flap tunneled under skin from back to front of mastectomy site. | Flap in place recreating breast contour with reconstructed nipple and areola |

This reconstruction procedure is typically performed when not enough fat and chest muscle is available to hold or cover an implant. During this procedure which takes several hours, the surgeon uses the latissimus dorsi, a back muscle, along with a section of skin and fat, to tunnel underneath the skin to the breast site to create a breast mound. An implant is then placed under the new chest muscle, with drains inserted to allow fluid that collects after surgery to drain out. The procedure leaves a scar on the back, in addition to the mastectomy scar on the front. Skin taken from the back may be a different color or texture. There may be an impairment of muscle power for some athletic activities due to the removal of the latissimus dorsi.(7)

Several weeks or months following the original surgery, depending on the patient's individual healing timetable, the nipple and areola construction can be surgically completed.

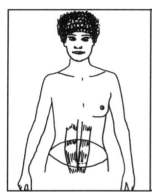

Two parallel rectus abdominus muscles with flap outlined.

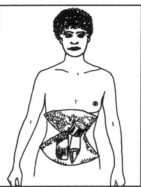

Flap of muscle, skin, and fat raised.

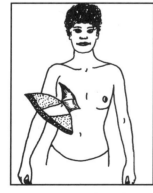

Flap tunneled under skin to mastectomy site.

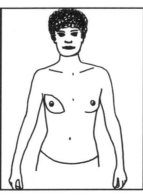

Flap in place recreating breast contour with reconstructed nipple and areola.

TRAM Flap (Transverse Rectus Abdominus Myocutaneous Flap Reconstruction)

This type of reconstruction may be used for women who are large-breasted, in addition to other reasons. The TRAM Flap is surgically performed by tunneling one of the two parallel vertical abdominal muscles (rectus abdominus muscles) up under the skin to the breast area along with enough skin and fat to create a breast mound. Taking the tissue and fat from the abdomen gives the result of a "tummy tuck," though there is a significant horizontal scar on the abdomen that remains,(3) in addition to the mastectomy scar on the chest. There is a possibility of weakness or hernia of the abdominal wall.(7)

Several weeks or months following the original surgery, depending on the patient's individual healing timetable, the nipple and areola construction can be surgically completed.

Free Flap Reconstruction

This surgical procedure is performed under general anesthesia by a plastic surgeon skilled in microsurgery, and takes anywhere from 9 to 12 hours. This technique involves taking a section of skin and fat from the abdomen, buttocks or thighs, and moving it unattached to the breast area, where the tiny blood vessels are reattached microscopically to recreate the blood flow which support healthy tissue. It takes great surgical skill, is more costly, and holds a higher risk of skin necrosis (skin death) due to the lack of blood support from the reattached blood vessels, but offers a very natural looking breast mound using the patient's own tissues, and, when successful, offers less over-all trauma to the body than either the Lats or TRAM Flap procedures.(1,5)

Sources: (1) *Breast Cancer,* by Yashar Hirshaut, M.D., F.A.C.P. and Peter I. Pressman, M.D., F.A.C.S.; (2) "Breast Reconstruction After Mastectomy," American Cancer Society #4630-PS, 1986; (3) "Breast Reconstruction, A Matter of Choice," National Cancer Institute #91-2151; (4) "Breast Reconstruction," by the American Society of Plastic and Reconstructive Surgeons, Inc. (5) *The Breast Cancer Companion,* by Kathy LaTour; (6) "Things You Should Know About Breast Reconstruction," by Dr. Richard A. Welk, Plastic Surgeon, The Polyclinic, Seattle, WA; (7) *Everyone's Guide to Cancer Therapy,* by Malin Dollinger, M.D., Ernest H. Rosenbaum, M.D., and Greg Cable. (8) Interview, Dr. Bruce Neu, Plastic Surgeon, Evergreen Hospital, Kirkland, WA; (9) Interview, Dr. Eric Taylor, Radiation Oncologist, Evergreen Hospital, Kirkland, WA.

Nipple and Areola Reconstruction

A new nipple and the areola (the darkened circular area around the nipple) can be reconstructed in a number a ways using small pieces of skin and fashioning both desired areas. Performed under either local or general anesthetic, the surgery typically lasts one to two hours. Flaps of the skin following reconstruction of the breast mound are raised to form the nipple. Skin for the areola may be taken from the other nipple (if large enough), lower abdomen, behind the ear, or in the groin, and then attached to the appropriate area. Tattooing is usually done "to achieve a good color match."(1) There are times when only the tattooing is done to create the illusion of a nipple presence. Tattooing is done under local anesthetic in the doctor's office.(1) The result, if done well, looks remarkably close to the original. Some women opt to have only the breast mound reconstructed, not the nipple and areola.

Sources: (1) *Breast Cancer: The Complete Guide,* by Yashar Hirshaut, M.D., F.A.C.P. and Peter I. Pressman, M.D., F.A.C.S.; (2) "Breast Reconstruction: A Matter of Choice," National Cancer Institute #91-2151; (3) "Breast Reconstruction After Mastectomy," American Cancer Society #6340-PS, 1986; (4) *Everyone's Guide to Cancer Therapy,* by Malin Dollinger, M.D., Ernest H. Rosenbaum, M.D., and Greg Cable; (5) *The Breast Cancer Companion,* by Kathy LaTour; (6) Interview, Dr. Bruce Neu, Plastic Surgeon, Evergreen Hospital, Kirkland, WA; (7) Interview, Dr. Richard Welk, Plastic Surgeon, The Polyclinic, Seattle, WA; (8) Interview, Dr. Thomas Johnson, Radiation Oncologist, and Kevin Belcher, Radiation Technician, Group Health Hospital, Seattle, WA; (9) Interview, Dr. Eric Taylor, Radiation Oncologist, Evergreen Hospital, Kirkland, WA.

ADJUVANT THERAPY

Adjuvant therapy is used to treat breast cancer following the removal of all known cancer by the use of surgery, when there is a high risk of hidden cancer cells somewhere in the body that could cause either a metastasis (cancer growth in another location), or recurrence of cancer in the same general area. Adjuvant therapy involves the use of anticancer drugs, such as chemotherapy, hormone (endocrine) therapy, and radiation treatment, with the intent of reducing the risk of recurrence, or prolonging survival.

ADJUVANT THERAPY CHOICES

With the increased sophistication and number of laboratory test results becoming available to oncologists, a highly individualized treatment is quite common.

Be aware that treatment recommendations are changing constantly with new information becoming available from ongoing research almost on a daily basis. It is an enormous challenge to a conscientious oncologist just to keep current. It is in the patient's best interest to request the most recent information available for her/his staging of breast cancer before agreeing to a course of treatment. It is the patient's life, after all.

It is quite appropriate to ask to view data currently available supporting treatment choices recommended, or where such data can be located. PDQ (Physicians Data Query) makes available to patients, doctors, and the public state-of-the-art choices for treatment of all types and stages of cancer. Simply call 1-800-4-CANCER for information.

Source: (1) "Adjuvant Therapy for Breast Cancer," American Cancer Society #5555.

NEO-ADJUVANT CHEMOTHERAPY

Combination chemotherapy (several anticancer drugs) is sometimes used, as is radiation therapy, to reduce the size of very large tumors before surgery.

CHEMOTHERAPY

Chemotherapy is the use of anticancer drugs in the treatment of cancer.

"When properly administered (they) will kill some normal cells, but not many...[C]ancer cells are much more sensitive to [chemotherapy drugs] than are normal cells. It is this difference in sensitivity that...we utilize to treat the cancer without injuring the patient."

— Yashar Hirshaut, M.D., F.A.C.P., *Breast Cancer*

There are four types of anticancer drugs being used as adjuvant therapy of breast cancer. They are:

1) *Alkylating Agents,* which damage the programs that control growth in the chromosomes of the tumor cells (e.g., Cytoxan (cyclophosphamide), Adriamycin (doxorubicin), and Thiotepa).

2) *Antimetabolites,* which interfere with the manufacture of nucleotides, the simple substances that make up DNA (e.g., Methotrexate and 5-Fluorouracil).

3) *Natural Products,* which interfere with cell structure and cell division, e.g., vincristine (Oncovin), and vinblastine (Velban), derived from the periwinkle plant.

4) *Hormones,* which affect the growth of breast cancer cells. Prednisone, related to cortisone, works to support the effects of other cytotoxic drugs. Tamoxifen (Nolvadex) works as an antiestrogen which, as a weak form of estrogen, interferes with the action of estrogen (which stimulates cancer growth), so inhibits tumor growth. Halotestin (fluoxymesterone), a male hormone, is sometimes used in hormone-receptive patients to inhibit tumor growth.

Source: (1) *Breast Cancer,* by Yashar Hirshaut, M.D., F.A.C.P. and Peter I. Pressman, M.D., F.A.C.S.

COMBINATION CHEMOTHERAPY

The following are common combinations of anticancer drugs used for the treatment of breast cancer. Very seldom is a single agent used currently, since there is much evidence to support that combination therapy is more successful.(1,2)

CMF: Cytoxan, methotrexate, and 5-fluorouracil (5-FU). Most common routine given due to its success rate for survival.

CAF: Cytoxan, Adriamycin, and 5-Fluorouracil (5-FU). Very common routine given for breast cancer.

FAC: 5-Fluorouracil (5-FU), Adriamycin, and Cytoxan. Similar to CAF, with higher doses of Adriamycin.

CAV: Cytoxan, Adriamycin, and vincristine. Typically used for more advanced disease, with lower doses of Adriamycin.

VATH: Vinblastine, Adriamycin, Thiotepa, Halotestin. Used when patients are at high risk for recurrence.

CMFVP: Vincristine and prednisone (or prednisolone) are added to CMF.

MF: Methotrexate and 5-Fluorouracil (5-FU) combined with leucovorin (folic acid). Has been found effective for women who are node negative.

Sources: (1) *Breast Cancer,* by Yashar Hirshaut, M.D., F.A.C.P. and Peter I. Pressman, M.D., F.A.C.S.; (2) "Chemotherapy and You," National Cancer Institute #92-1136.

ADMINISTRATION OF CHEMOTHERAPY

Depending on the type and availability of drugs, the doctor and/or clinic's preference, the staging of breast cancer, and the patient's response to the drugs, chemotherapy may be given 1) orally, in pill, capsule, or liquid form; 2) topically, applied to the skin; 3) intramuscularly, directly into a cancerous area in the skin by the injection of a needle; 4) intravenously (IV), inserted through a thin needle into a vein, usually on the hand, or lower arm. A catheter can also be used, which is a thin tube placed into a large vein in the body, and remaining there the duration of treatment for easier and less debilitating access to the veins. Also called "venous access devices." Ask your doctor for the options available to you for treatment. Call the American Cancer Society (1-800-ACS-2345) for more specific information.

Sources: (1) *Breast Cancer,* by Yashar Hirshaut, M.D., F.A.C.P. and Peter I. Pressman, M.D., F.A.C.S.; (2) "Chemotherapy and You," National Cancer Institute #92-1136.

SIDE EFFECTS

Some people take chemotherapy with no noticeable side effects. The most common side effects, when they do occur, are: nausea, fatigue, hair loss, weight gain, white blood cell and platelet count drop, phlebitis, acid stomach, temporary arthritis, menopausal symptoms (sweating, hot flashes, and mood swings), menstrual changes, and fertility effects. The side effects specific to a broader spectrum of anticancer drugs used in breast cancer treatment are given in the anticancer drug section following.

Anticancer drugs go after any cell that quickly divides, which is typical of a cancer cell. Some normal body cells also divide quickly, so may be targeted by the drugs used, as well: hair (alopecia—hair loss), bone marrow, cells of the mouth (stomatitis) and skin, as well as stomach and intestinal cells.

SUGGESTION: *Keep track on a notepad the type of drugs, and dosages given, and your reactions to them at each chemo session. This will assist the doctor in adjusting the dosages (or supporting you with available drugs that may offset some of the negative symptoms) for your comfort during treatment when possible.*

— Marie Baker, breast cancer warrior

Hair Loss

"This is the side effect that causes women the greatest sadness. At a time when they are extremely vulnerable, their appearance may be radically changed, and their illness given a visible and very upsetting public manifestation...But...every strand of hair will grow back."(1)

Not all chemotherapy will cause hair loss. However some chemotherapy agents, such as Adriamycin, are more likely than others to cause the loss of hair.

If hair loss does occur, it can affect all parts of the body, including arms, legs, underarms, the pubic area, as well as the head, eyebrows, and eyelashes.(3) To reduce the trauma of gradual hair loss, with hair falling everywhere—"on my pillow, in the tub, on my clothes, in the sink, in food"(2)—some people choose to cut their hair short or have a friend or loved one shave their head prior to treatment.(3)

If your doctor says hair loss is likely with the chemotherapy treatment, select a wig or two *before* going into treatment. If finances are a concern, call the American Cancer Society, 1-800-ACS-2345, which has used wigs available free of charge for cancer patients. Some insurance companies cover wig costs if a doctor writes a prescription for a "cranial prosthesis."(2) Caps, turbans, and scarves are excellent alternatives to a wig.(3)

Check into the possibility of attending "Look Good—Feel Better" classes through the American Cancer Society, which teach makeup application, wig styling, the use of scarves, and how to buy lingerie to those going through cancer.(2) Or read *Beauty and Cancer,* by Diane Noyes, for assistance in dealing with the aspects of attractiveness during treatment.

Call the American Cancer Society, 1-800-ACS-2345, or the National Cancer Institute, 1-800-4-CANCER, for the latest information available on hair loss.

SUGGESTIONS: To keep as much hair as possible, with the least amount of hair damage: use a gentle shampoo, and shampoo less frequently. Use a wide-toothed comb to untangle hair instead of a brush, and instead of using hair dryers and curling irons, try air drying and using styling gel or spray.(2)

SCALP TOURNIQUETS AND ICE CAPS(4)

Scalp tourniquets and *ice caps* were used prior to 1990 in an attempt to prevent or reduce hair loss. In reviewing their safety and effectiveness, the Food and Drug Administration (FDA) became concerned regarding the lack of supportive clinical evidence for their use, so halted their manufacturer. The FDA had the following concerns:

1) The potential for *scalp metastasis* posed by the use of these devices;

2) The potential for *reducing drug circulation to other anatomic sites beyond the scalp,* such as the skull and possibly the brain; and

3) *The effectiveness of these devices in preventing hair loss* and *how specific cytologic doses and other variables affected the results achieved.*

The manufacturers did not come forward with data supporting their safety and effectiveness, so they are no longer being manufactured in the United States.

Sources: (1) *Breast Cancer,* by Yashar Hirshaut, M.D., F.A.C.P. and Peter I. Pressman, M.D., F.A.C.S.; (2) *The Breast Cancer Companion,* by Kathy LaTour; (3) *The Breast Cancer Handbook,* by Joan Swirsky and Barbara Balaban; (4) *Cancer: Principles and Practice of Oncology.* 4th ed. by Vincent T. DeVita, Jr., M.D., Samuel Hellerman, M.D., and Steven A. Rosenberg, M.D., Ph.D.; J.B. Lippincott, 1993.

WHAT IS CHEMOTHERAPY ABLE TO ACHIEVE?

- Cures cancer.
- Keeps the cancer from spreading.
- Slows cancer's growth.
- Relieves symptoms that may be caused by the cancer.

Source: (1) "Chemotherapy," American Cancer Society; "Chemotherapy and You," National Cancer Institute #92-1136.

ANTICANCER DRUGS

Adrenocorticosteroids (Prednisone) (Decadron)
How Administered: Oral, Intravenous, Intramuscular.
Side Effects: Could lead to peptic ulcer or pancreatitis, edema (fluid and salt retention), headaches, sleeplessness, vertigo, psychiatric problems, muscle weakness (low potassium), osteoporosis, bone damage to hips, increased hair growth, increased blood sugar (diabetes), cataracts, malaise, increased infections.

Adriamycin, *see* Doxorubicin.

Adrucil, *see* 5-Fluorouracil.

Androgens (Testosterone)/Fluoxymesterone (Halotestin)
How Administered: Oral, Intramuscular.
Side Effects: Loss of menstrual periods, masculinization, hoarseness, acne, clitoral enlargement, increased hair growth, jaundice, leg swelling (edema), nausea, intestinal upset, fluid and mineral imbalance.

Cyclophosphamide (Cytoxan)
How Administered: Oral, Intravenous.
Side Effects: Bladder irritation, blood in urine, liver problems, fever, chills, anemia, low blood counts, joint pains, swollen feet, slow blood clotting, vomiting, loss of hair, dizziness, confusion, infertility, second malignancy, headache, mouth sores, diarrhea, gastrointestinal ulcers, skin darkening.

Cytoxan, *see* Cyclophosphamide.

Doxorubicin (Adriamycin)
How Administered: Intravenous.
Side Effects: Hair loss, anemia, low blood counts, fever, chills, diarrhea, vomiting, bleeding, risk of infection, red urine (not bloody), very low white blood cell counts, skin cracking, sore mouth, iron loss, loss of appetite, shortness of breath.

Estrogens (Diethylstilbestrol)(DES)

Used for breast metastases (women five or more years postmenopausal and receptor positive).

How Administered: Oral.

Side Effects: Increased clotting, enlarged breast, testicle atrophy, loss of libido, edema (fluid retention), water-soluble vitamin deficiency, iron deficiency, gall stones, sugar intolerance, increased serum calcium, constipation, loss of appetite, nausea, vomiting.

Fluorouracil (5-FU)

How Administered: Intravenous, Oral, Topical.

Side Effects: Rash, sun rash, rare heart toxicity, hair loss, vomiting, diarrhea, fever, chills, low blood counts, skin darkening, nail cracking and loss, eye irritation, sore mouth and throat.

Interferon-alpha/Intron-A/Roferon-A

How Administered: Intramuscular, Subcutaneous.

Side Effects: Fever, chills, joint pain, low blood counts, fever, fatigue, weight loss, sweating, dizziness, rash, vomiting, sore mouth, diarrhea, altered taste and smell

Leucovorin (Folinic acid)

Used to reverse toxic reactions to methotrexate, and to increase effectiveness of 5-FU.

How Administered: Oral, Intramuscular, Intravenous.

Side Effects: Allergic reactions, vomiting, nausea, anemic symptoms.

Megesterol

How Administered: Oral.

Side Effects: Vein inflammation, hair loss, fluid retention, problem pregnancy.

Melphalan (Alkeran)

How Administered: Oral.

Side Effects: Low blood counts, second malignancies, pulmonary scarring, loss of menstrual periods, dermatitis, nausea, vomiting, sore mouth, increased uric acid.

Methotrexate (Mexate)

How Administered: Oral, Intravenous, Intramuscular, Subcutaneous, Spinal (intrathecal).

Side Effects: Nausea, vomiting, diarrhea, loss of appetite, mouth sores, stomach pain, risk of infection, slow blood clotting, low blood counts, skin rash, lung scarring, shortness of breath, seizures, dizziness, kidney and liver problems, sensitivity to sunlight.

Mitomycin-C (Mutamycin)

How Administered: Intravenous.

Side Effects: Vomiting, diarrhea, fever, chills, mouth sores, bleeding, blood in urine, kidney problems, second malignancy, sores at site of injection, risk of infection, hair loss, loss of appetite, slow blood clotting.

Mitoxantrone (Novantrone)

How Administered: Intravenous.

Side Effects: Low blood counts, skin bruises, fatigue, nausea, vomiting, diarrhea, heart problems, mouth sores, risk of infection, fever, lung problems, headaches, seizures, hair loss, bleeding, urine may turn green.

Progestins (Megace, Provera)

How Administered: Oral, Intramuscular.

Side Effects: Vaginal bleeding, spotting and change in menstrual cycle, lack of menstrual periods, edema, jaundice, allergic rash, itching, nausea, vomiting, weight gain, mental depression.

Tamoxifen (Nolvadex)

How Administered: Oral.

Side Effects: Hot flashes, vaginal bleeding, mood swings, bone pain, fluid retention, itching, nausea, vomiting, taste changes, high calcium levels in the blood, problem pregnancy, increased risk for endometrial (uterine) cancer, possible risk of liver cancer (rare).

Taxol

How Administered: Intravenous.

Side Effects: Low blood counts, hair loss, sores in mouth and throat, muscle and joint pain, numbness, difficulty moving, allergic reactions.

ThioTEPA (Triethylenethiophosphoramide)

How Administered: Intravenous, Intracavitary.

Side Effects: Low blood counts, headaches, fever, dizziness, bronchoconstriction, local pain, loss of appetite, nausea, vomiting, potential secondary malignancies, anemia, bleeding, infection, birth defects.

Velban, *see* Vinblastine.

Vinblastine (Velban)

How Administered: Intravenous.

Side Effects: Nausea, vomiting, pain at IV site if drug leaks, risk of infection, hair loss, low blood counts, peripheral neuropathies, headache, rash, anorexia, sore mouth or throat, constipation, abdominal discomfort, nervous system problems, fever, chills, jaw pain, infertility.

Vincristine (Oncovin)

How Administered: Intravenous.

Side Effects: Severe reaction with IV leak, numbness, low blood count, constipation, difficulty walking, hair loss, headache, jaw pain, joint pain, weakness, dry mouth, nervous system problems, difficult urination, fever, chills, sore throat, mouth sores, bleeding, infertility, altered taste and smell.

NOTE: *This section's format is taken in large part from* Everyone's Guide to Cancer Therapy, *by Malin Dollinger, M.D., F.A.C.P., Ernest H. Rosenbaum, M.D., F.A.C.S., and Greg Cable.*

Hormones and Antihormones(2)

Adrenocorticoids (cortisone-like), Prednisone, Decadron (Hexadrol), Medrol

Side Effects: Increased appetite, sense of well-being, sleeplessness (insomnia) and agitation, fluid retention and weight gain, diabetes, high blood pressure, increased risk of infection, acne-like risk of infection, stomach and intestinal ulcers, loss of potassium, muscle weakness, cramps, or pain, increased hair growth (hirsutism), decreased or blurry vision, frequent urination, mood changes, menstrual problems, sterility, irregular heart beat, osteoporosis (weakening of bones).

Androgens ("male hormones"), Halotestin, Depo-testosterone, Deca-Durabolin, Flutamide (Eulexin)

Side Effects: Nausea, vomiting, liver problems, lowering of voice, skin changes, water retention and weight gain, changes in libido, constipation, diarrhea, bladder problems, changes in menstruation, hot flashes, itchy and burning vagina.

Antiestrogens, Tamoxifen (Nolvadex), Nafodide

Side Effects: Nausea, vomiting, hot flashes, loss of appetite, vaginal discharge, itching, bleeding, headache, blurred vision, confusion, weakness, sleepiness, increased fertility, bone pain, pain or swelling in legs, skin rash, weight gain, shortness of breath.

Estrogens ("female hormones"), DES (diethylstilbestrol), Stilphostrol, Tace, Estradiol

Side Effects: Nausea, vomiting, fluid retention and weight gain, swollen and tender breasts, headache, dizziness, depression, lethargy, lowered blood calcium, heart and circulation problems, worsening of nearsightedness or astigmatism, difficulty wearing contact lenses, abdominal cramps, diarrhea, constipation, changes in menstruation, sterility, loss of potassium, vaginal infections, cervical secretions, skin changes, excess body hair.

232 ~ *Stealing the Dragon's Fire*

Progestogens, Delalutin, Depo-Provera, Medroxyprogesterone

Side Effects: Fluid retention, weight gain, nausea, vomiting, abdominal cramps, dizziness, headache, lethargy, depression, heart and circulatory problems, changes in menstruation, cervical secretions, vaginal infections, decreased libido, skin rash, breast enlargement or tenderness.

Megace (Megesterolacetate)

Side Effects: Fluid retention, weight gain, increased fat deposits, hair loss or thinning, liver damage, fatigue, nausea, vomiting, carpal tunnel syndrome.

Biological Response Modifiers(2)

CSF (Colony-Stimulating Factor): Colony-stimulating factors are substances that are normally produced by the body to help the bone marrow cells to develop. To restore bone marrow more quickly after chemotherapy, laboratories are also manufacturing CSF. Therefore, higher doses of chemotherapy may be given more safely.

IFN (Interferon): Alpha-interferon first became known for its antiviral abilities but soon was noted for its anticancer properties. Interferon has varied effectiveness, and it continues to be tested.

IL (Interleukin): Interleukin transmits signals between leukocytes (white blood cells). Some interleukins have been shown to fight cancer.

MAbs (Monoclonal Antibodies): Monoclonal Antibodies are bits of protein that can locate and bind to tumor cells in the body. It can be used alone to detect or eliminate tumors, or they may be linked to drugs, toxins, or radioactive material, which they carry directly to cancer cells, avoiding healthy cells.

TNF (Tumor Necrosis Factor): Tumor necrosis factor acts as a chemical messenger between cells, triggering immune defenses that destroy tumors. Testing has shown that animals with cancer can no longer produce their own TNF.

Sources: (1) *Everyone's Guide To Cancer Therapy,* by Malin Dollinger, M.D., Ernest H. Rosenbaum, M.D., and Greg Cable; (2) *Coping with Chemotherapy* by Nancy Bruning; (3) *The Facts About Chemotherapy,* by Paul R. Reich, M.D.

HORMONE THERAPY

Hormone therapy is a form of chemical therapy which utilizes a drug that reduces hormones or affects their interaction with cancer cells. Currently, the most commonly used hormone treatment is tamoxifen (Nolvadex), an antiestrogen, or estrogen block.

Tamoxifen is most commonly described as blocking the estrogen receptors, which, when they receive the body's estrogen, have the ability to encourage cancer growth. When tamoxifen blocks the reception of estrogen, it is thought to short-circuit this process, and seems to prevent recurrence of breast cancer at that site. There are alternate theories of just how tamoxifen works chemically, such as cell starvation, neutralizing a cancer-causing enzyme, and others. The important thing for the patient is that it appears to be very effective at arresting cancer growth in the breast, so a marked decrease in both local recurrences and second unrelated cancers is noted. It may also have "mildly protective effects on bones and the circulatory system."(6) There are relatively few known side effects for most women, compared to other chemotherapy agents.

Clinical studies show that postmenopausal women with cancerous breasts, involved lymph nodes, and no metastasis, in addition to postmenopausal women with negative nodes, show increased survival rates with adjuvant hormone treatment, though premenopausal women do not respond to such treatment, but rather do better with chemotherapy, according to Dr. Paul Reich.(5)

The typical tamoxifen dosage is 20 mg a day, taken orally in the form of two pills, morning and evening. It is recommended that a woman stay on tamoxifen for anywhere from two to five years, to a lifetime, states oncologist Dr. Mukund Sargur.

Hormone treatment is now being offered as a combined treatment with chemotherapy due to its apparent ability to stave off recurrence.

Eligible for Hormone Therapy? An estrogen receptor assay is done to determine if a patient's breast cancer cells removed during surgery have receptors on them. Estrogen receptors are believed to bind the female hormone, estrogen, which is believed to encourage cancer growth. Tumors with these receptors are more likely to respond to hormone therapy to inhibit cancer cell growth. Most post-menopausal women have positive receptors, and respond well to hormone treatment.(5)

Financial Assistance: The Patient Assistance Program (PAP) was developed by ICI Pharmaceuticals to supply Nolvadex free of charge, (due to its high cost) to those patients who otherwise could not afford it. Call 1-800-456-5678, ext. 2592, for more information.

Side Effects: Most common: hot flashes, night sweats, vaginal dryness, and mood swings, including depression (menopausal symptoms). Less common: blurred vision, nausea, breast tenderness and swelling, bone pain, bloating, possible birth defects if a woman becomes pregnant while taking it (does not prevent pregnancy).(6) A few patients, particularly those whose cancer has spread to the bone, are known to show an increased supply of calcium in the blood, which can be dangerous, so blood tests need to be done when treatment begins.(5) Recent research indicates an increased incidence of endometrial (lining of the uterus) cancer, and possible rare development of liver cancer (with high doses of tamoxifen—40 mg/day), for those who take tamoxifen.

Call the National Cancer Institute for free publications on the most up-to-date information on tamoxifen treatment.
1-800-4-CANCER.

RADIATION THERAPY

Radiation therapy is a treatment that uses X-rays to kill cancer cells locally in a cancer-affected area. It most often follows a lumpectomy to insure a cancer-free area. Radiation may be used when cancer has been located near the chest wall, to irradiate the edges of tissue that remain after breast cancer is surgically removed, or at the location of a metastatic site, such as the bone. At times radiation is used to decrease the size of a large tumor before surgery to reduce the amount of breast tissue removed at the time of surgery, or as a combined treatment with chemotherapy (before, in the middle, or at the end) and/or surgery to increase the probability of a total cure. For example, if a large tumor is reduced significantly by irradiation, the surgeon may be able to perform a lumpectomy rather than a mastectomy at the time of surgery, or the choice and/or extent of chemotherapy might be altered.

Radiation is also used to slow the growth, or reduce pressure, bleeding, pain or other symptoms (palliative treatment) of an advanced or metastatic cancer by reducing the tumor size at a particular location.

MEDICAL TEAM

Radiation Oncologist: A doctor who specializes in using radiation to treat disease.

Radiation Technologist (Therapist): A person with special training who runs the equipment that delivers the radiation.

Dosimetrist: a person who plans and calculates the proper radiation dose for treatment.

EQUIPMENT

The linear accelerator is currently the most commonly used X-ray machine for radiation treatment of breast cancer in accredited facilities. It is a high energy, deeply penetrating, intricately computed and managed beam of X-ray delivered to the patient in regulated doses five days a week over a matter of weeks, most typically for breast cancer, 5½ to 6½ weeks. The linear accelerator, as opposed to the older cobalt machines, produces less skin irritation during treatment, though some acute irritation and eventual tissue thickening is usually noted.

Those patients who have a lumpectomy will usually get an electron beam boost at the end of their treatment, which provides a higher dose to the surgical site ("tumor bed") to kill any lingering cancer cells. Some doctors will use a radiation implant instead; tubes surgically placed at the lumpectomy site are filled with radioactive material, which then emit the prescribed dosage over a period of time. The patient is hospitalized during the implant. This procedure is no longer commonly used, since the electron beam boost procedure offers the patient less pain, discomfort, and inconvenience, at a lesser medical cost.

TREATMENT

"Precision in set-up assures radiation delivered with a high degree of accuracy to the sites of concern. There is very little scatter of X-rays elsewhere in the body—but some." Special shields, if used, would not work, since "one cannot shield effectively high energy radiation from a linear accelerator."
Dr. Thomas Johnson, Radiation Oncologist, Seattle, WA

A visit with the radiation oncologist is the first step in radiation treatment, when the doctor goes over the planned routine with the patient. This provides an excellent opportunity for the patient to ask questions or address any particular concerns.

Next, a *"simulation" appointment,* or appointments, are made. During "simulation," very exacting calculations are computed. *Pen* and/or *tattoo markings* are made on the skin to map out the exact locations where the beams of X-ray will be directed.

The *tattoo* is a permanent marking which is used so that 1) the exact locations for dosage entry are not lost during treatment, and 2) should radiation treatment be needed in the future, the previous exposure site will be clearly defined. (This is important, since each body area has an upper limit for X-ray exposure that is considered safe.) If the patient prefers pen markings, the request needs to be addressed to the radiation oncologist. The "simulation" appointments, which may take two hours or more, require patience on the part of the patient, who must lie very still as these calculations and markings are made on the body surface, the accuracy of which is essential for the safest, most effective treatment.

Then *daily treatments* begin, Monday through Friday. The treatment machine delivers the prescribed dose in a few minutes, but the patient is in the room being correctly positioned for 10 to 20 minutes. Depending on the tumor, treatment will be delivered to the area of breast considered at risk. The armpit (axillary lymph nodes) is included if there was lymph node involvement. Radiation Oncologist Dr. Thomas Johnson indicates that they no longer treat axilla if only one node is involved and the node has not been replaced by tumor (extracapsular extension). Standard dosage is about 5,900 to 6,400 rads ("radiation absorbed dose"), with daily dosages of about 180 to 200 units per day.(4) A woman may feel somewhat claustrophobic lying under the radiation machine. Speaking directly to the radiation technologist or oncologist is appropriate, so they can assist the patient in feeling comfortable.

Reduced-field, or electron beam boost treatment is then usually given to the surgical site if a lumpectomy was performed, to insure the killing of any remaining cancer cells. This is given as an electron beam dosage of about 1,600 to 2,000 rads over five to seven days. The 1,600 to 2,000 rads are usually included in the total count of 5,900 to 6,400 rads of 'standard dosage,' according to Dr. Thomas Johnson.

SIDE EFFECTS

1) *Skin irritation:* itching or burning (sometimes blistering with more severe reactions), usually noted towards the end of the treatment cycle. The extent varies from patient to patient. It is important to use only doctor-recommended creams to relieve the symptoms, since home remedies or over-the-counter lotions

may increase irritation and/or interfere with the radiation. Lotions recommended may be emollients, such as aloe vera or Vitamin E cream. Topical steroids may be prescribed;

2) *fatigue:* the amount may vary from patient to patient, and may be due to the stress (as much as by the actual treatment) created by the effort required to rearrange one's life around daily radiation appointments;

3) *changes in the skin:* sensitivity, particularly to heat for several months, darkening, enlargement of pores, and thickening or firmness of the breast tissue (fibrosis)(4);

4) *sensitivity of the treated area to sunlight:* during treatment and for about one year following, the patient should take precautions, such as sunscreens, when out in the sunlight;

5) some women complain of a *dry cough* or a *lump in the throat, discomfort in the breasts* following treatment, *increased sensitivity to rib injury,* and *scarring* from severe X-ray burning (rare).

DANGER OF RECURRENCE DUE TO X-RAY TREATMENT

According to the National Cancer Institute, there is a chance of local recurrence in the irradiated breast, particularly for women under 35 years of age. However, overall survival rates for both 1) the mastectomy treatment and 2) the lumpectomy plus radiation treatment has been found to be equivalent. ("Breast Cancer," *PDQ Information,* 12/5/94.)

Current doses of X-ray are much more carefully administered than in the past due to the advancements available to the doctor by the *linear accelerator.* However, a patient needs to address any particular concerns to the radiation oncologist, who should have available the most current information regarding the issues of safety at the time of treatment.

For the most effective treatment, and to insure maximum safety to the patient, it is important to be sure the patient facility using X-ray is accredited and the radiation oncologist is board-certified.

Call the American Cancer Society for information on accredited facilities, and board-certified radiation oncologists in your area.

Personal Resources: Thomas Johnson, M.D., Radiation Oncologist and Kevin Belcher, Radiation Technician, Group Health Hospital, Seattle, WA; Eric Taylor, M.D., Radiation Oncologist, Evergreen Hospital, Kirkland, WA.; Mukund Sargur, M.D., Oncologist, Hematologist, Internist, Evergreen Hospital, Kirkland, WA; Judith Jones, Cancer Information Specialist, Evergreen Cancer Center, Kirkland, WA; Oncology Staff and Consenting Patients, Oncology Department, Evergreen Cancer Center, Evergreen Hospital, Kirkland, WA.

Sources: (1) *Choice In Cancer: Integrating the Best of Conventional and Alternative Approaches to Cancer,* by Michael Lerner, Ph.D.; (2) *Coping With Chemotherapy,* by Nancy Bruning; (3) *Everyone's Guide to Cancer Therapy,* by Malin Dollinger, M.D., Ernest H. Rosenbaum, M.D., and Greg Cable; (4) *The Breast Cancer Companion,* by Kathy LaTour; (5) *The Facts About Chemotherapy,* by Paul R. Reich, M.D.; (6) *Women's Cancers,* by Kerry A. McGinn, R.N., and Pamela J. Haylock, R.N.

Pamphlets: "Radiation Therapy and You," U.S. Department of Health and Human Services, available through National Cancer Institute. "Radiation Therapy," U.S. Department of Health and Human Services, also available through National Cancer Institute.

For the most up-to-date, and more detailed information on Hormone Therapy, Chemotherapy, and Radiation therapy, call the American Cancer Society at 1-800-ACS-2345, or the National Cancer Institute at 1-800-4-CANCER.

BONE-MARROW OR STEM-CELL TRANSPLANT COMBINED WITH HIGH-DOSE CHEMOTHERAPY

High-dose chemotherapy is used occasionally for patients with advanced-stage breast cancer combined with bone-marrow or stem-cell transplantation when only a slim possibility of survival is available, and, after much testing, it is determined that the patient is a good candidate for this treatment. It has recently become available for breast cancer patients with more than 10 lymph nodes involved, though it is a very high-risk treatment with data for survival still being collected.

Ultra-high doses of chemotherapy are administered to the patient, "so large that they destroy not only cancer cells, but normal bone-marrow cells, as well,"(2) and sometimes radiation, to kill all malignant cells in the body.

The patient is then "rescued" by the infusion of healthy bone marrow, or peripheral blood stem cells, to re-establish a healthy blood cell system.

Before chemotherapy treatment, the patient's bone marrow, or stem cells, are extracted and stored. After chemotherapy treatment is over, the bone marrow, or the stem cells, are replaced into the blood-stream of the body in an effort to encourage the body to begin the healthy replacement of healthy blood cells. The current use of colony stimulating factors, drugs that encourage the redevelopment of healthy blood cells, are now used to hasten the recovery of the body from the toxic effects of high-dose chemotherapy, which essentially destroys the body's ability to defend itself against infection.

Bone marrow is the spongy tissue located inside bones that produces the body's blood cells, including white blood cells (leukocytes), infection fighters; red blood cells (erythrocytes), those which carry oxygen to and removed waste products from organs and tissues, and platelets, which allow the blood to clot.(1)

AUTOLOGOUS TRANSPLANTATION

This involves the *extracting, storing,* and then *transplanting* (replacing) *of the patient's own bone marrow, or peripheral blood stem cells, combined with a treatment of high-dose chemotherapy.* Autologous is preferred over a donor transplant: allogeneic, (marrow from a sibling or a tissue match), or syngeneic (marrow from an identical twin) when possible, to reduce the risk of graft-versus-host-disease (GVHD), or graft rejection, which can be life-threatening.

BONE-MARROW TRANSPLANTATION

This type of transplantation involves:
1) *the harvest of the desired amount of bone marrow* (1-2 quarts of marrow and blood, about 2 percent of the body's bone marrow);
2) *a treatment of high-dose, toxic chemotherapy and/or radiation* in an attempt to kill all cancer cells present in any stage, plus any diseased bone marrow, at the time of treatment; and
3) *the replacement of the patient's own bone marrow* (transplant) responsible for the development of healthy blood cells in the body combined with treatment with colony stimulating factors (e.g., GM-CSF, or G-CSF), with the hope that the body can replenish a full supply of healthy blood cells and the ability to ward off infection or disease, typical of a state of health. The two to four weeks following transplantation is critical, a time of waiting while the body is at great risk for infection, until the body demonstrates with the blood count that the transplant has been accepted by the body.

PERIPHERAL BLOOD STEM-CELL TRANSPLANTATION

Instead of extracting and replacing the body's bone marrow, as described above, the peripheral (circulating) blood stem cells are used. The procedure:

1) First, a *colony growth stimulator* (e.g., GM-CSF, or G-CSF) *is injected into the stem cell donor* (patient) over a period of a few days;

2) *The growth factors are given time to stimulate the growth of the peripheral blood stem cells*, and then released into the blood stream;

3) *The stem cells are then collected from the donor's (patient's) blood, and stored frozen* until the high doses of chemotherapy have been completed. Collection is done by a technique called *leukapheresis,* which circulates the blood through a filtering process, using a centrifuge to separate out different blood products by their specific gravities. The patient is simply hooked up to an IV during the procedure. The blood products separated out for transplantation are the white blood cells and peripheral blood stem cells. The rest of the blood is then returned to the patient.

   The peripheral (circulating) stem cells are called "seed" cells, from which all of the body's specialized blood cells develop. Stem cells are normally produced in the bone marrow, but are also found circulating through the blood system; they form the building blocks of the the immune and blood systems;

4) *Once the stem cells are harvested and stored, high-dose chemotherapy is administered;*

5) *Once this therapy is completed, the stored white blood cells and stem cells are thawed and replaced (transplanted) into the patient's blood stream by an IV.* After this begins the *waiting time* to see if the treatment has been effective.

"The revived white cells go right to work fighting infection, and the stem cells find their way to key sectors of the patient's bones and begin reconstituting the marrow to produce more blood cells of every type."(3)

Dr. William Bensinger, head of the team of doctors at Fred Hutchinson Cancer Research Center (Seattle, WA) studying this procedure, states that both the white cells and the stem cells come back a number of days sooner than found in bone marrow transplants, which translates into less likelihood of "serious infections or blood complication...The initial success of stem cell transplantation offers new hope for treating...breast cancers,"(3) and better support for intensive dose chemotherapy or radiation treatment.

Transplantation is a treatment being offered to women with high-risk, later-staged breast cancer as a possible alternative. However, the patient needs to be fully aware of the risks involved for treatment. Talk to your doctor, and/or call the National Cancer Institute for more information regarding transplantation, and available facilities for transplantation in your area: 1-800-4-CANCER.

Sources: (1) *Bone Marrow Transplants,* edited by Susan K. Steward; (2) *Mobilization of Peripheral Blood Stem Cells for Support of High- Dose Chemotherapy Protocols at Swedish Medical Center,* by Erin D. Ellis, M.D., Gary E. Goodman, M.D., Henry G. Kaplan, M.D., et al; (3) "Transplanting Bone Marrow—Without Transplanting Marrow," *Quest* [a quarterly publication by Fred Hutchinson Cancer Research Center Seattle, WA], Fall 1993; (4) Interview, Erin D. Ellis, M.D., Swedish Tumor Institute, Seattle, WA.

ALTERNATIVE TREATMENTS

For the individual diagnosed with breast cancer, the question of what type of treatment will best insure survival can be piercing. The most predictable success for the cancer patient (from present research available) is to take the standard treatment offered (surgery, chemotherapy, radiation, hormone treatment). In addition, it is believed that patients combine unique personal choices of complementary therapies, which reflect a wide spectrum of personal and cultural choices that seek to honor the whole body.(2) These might be anything—diet changes or vitamin additives, cultural medicines such as Chinese herbs, physical activities such as tai chi or yoga, visual imagery, drumming, chanting, creating art, praying, or deep meditation, and many more. It is believed that as many as a half or more of present cancer patients may use some type of complementary therapy to increase their odds for survival and/or quality of life during treatment.

According to Michael Lerner, *"...the starting point for informed choice in both mainstream and complementary cancer therapies is the patient's recognition that he can play a crucial role in the fight for his life. [This] reaches beyond choices about therapy to choices about how we intend to live each day for the rest of our lives."*(2)

There are those who opt to seek treatment outside standard medical treatment either because of personal preference and/or choice, dissatisfaction with medical personnel and/or treatment, knowledge of other options or unusual successes, or perhaps, fear. There are those who choose no treatment at all.

It is important to note that there is much international variation in treating cancer. According to Dr. Lerner in *Choice In Cancer,* a compendium of knowledge available regarding complementary and alternative treatment choices, cancer treatment as practiced in the United States may be considered quite harsh by medical personnel elsewhere in the world as compared to treatments offered in their countries, which often use less radical treatment choices, and more varied combined treatment plans which seek to support the body's capabilities to regain health in different ways than is normally supported medically and insurance-wise here in the United States.

The American Cancer Society (1-800-ACS-2345) has available a printed copy of the risks and dangers it suggests a patient takes when choosing treatment options outside standard treatment options currently being offered in the United States, as well as a list of alternative treatments that they consider questionable. It is important for the patient to be aware that there are treatments being offered cancer patients for quite substantial sums of money that have not been proven effective medically or scientifically as cancer treatments, that may be staffed by unqualified medical staff, and that may offer surgical or medical treatment that may be harmful, even fatal. Cancer provides occasions where the patient and/or loved ones may feel desperate for a solution, a cure. Be aware that there are those who may be willing to take advantage of such desperation.

Cautions Regarding Alternative Treatments

- Be thoroughly informed on any treatment you are considering and its track record with individual patients. Ask to speak with patients.
- Insist on well-qualified medical personnel. Check their credentials.
- Be very cautious of a treatment program that insists you drop all others to be on theirs.
- Ask for available literature on treatment offered. Check it out at the library, or by calling 1-800-4-CANCER.(1)

There are clinical trials available to patients who wish to try new treatments. Call 1-800-4-CANCER for more information.

SUGGESTION: *Take your time to make treatment choices. If you feel you are being rushed, you may want to get a second opinion, or even a third. If you decide to combine complementary treatments with the standard treatment you are taking, consult with your doctor. Some combinations may work against each other, others may enhance treatment. Doctors are becoming more aware of patients making these choices, and will probably be supportive as long as your choices enhance treatment, or your quality of life.*

"So when all the information is before you, consider turning inward to discover from as deep a source as possible: WHAT MAKES SENSE TO YOU?"

— Dr. Michael Lerner, *Choice In Cancer*

Sources: (1) *Charting the Journey,* (NCCS), edited by Fitzhugh Mullan, M.D., Barbara Hoffman, J.D., and editors of Consumer Reports Books; (2) *Choice In Cancer,* by Michael Lerner. Ph.D.; (3) "General Information on Questionable Methods of Cancer Treatment," American Cancer Society #8249.

OPTIONS

"I believe that people who are inclined to fight for life with cancer using whatever combination of conventional and complementary cancer therapies that makes sense to them are wise to do so."

— Dr. Michael Lerner, *Choice In Cancer*

There is increasing interest in the medical and scientific arena of what might be available for fighting the disease of cancer combining different kinds of effective treatment. Dr. Lerner's book, *Choice In Cancer,* is an enormous compendium of information made available to the public, gathered as a result of many years of being involved in Commonweal, a health and environmental research institute in Bolinas, California, interfacing with patients with cancer and the medical community, attempting to address the many issues surrounding this disease. He explores international variations in cancer treatment, spiritual, psychological, nutritional, vitamin and mineral supplements, plus integrated therapies such as nutritional, and immunotherapy programs. Physical exercise, massage, therapeutic touch, chiropractic, traditional Chinese medicines, and still other more unconventional types of treatment are offered in an open arena of inquiry. It is an outstanding source of information available for exploring the available treatments in treating serious disease.

According to Lerner, it is very common for cancer patients to be using traditional cultural, or folk, medicines in combination with standard western medical treatments, whether or not they identify this to the medical community with whom they are interfacing. Chinese herbal medicines and acupuncture are good examples of this, as is tai chi, a kind of traditional meditational pattern of exercise which is believed to help balance the energies of the body, and therefore support its emerging health. Music, relaxation techniques, meditation, prayer, humor, art, vitamin supplements, and exercise regimens—the list goes on. There are possibly as many alternative forms of attempting to support good health as there are different cultures, and then, given the variations found within each culture, perhaps multiplied many times. In many countries around the world, folk medicines are supported as part of the valued treatment of a patient trying to regain his health.(1) Lerner asserts that Western medicine is considered the most harsh to the body by medical communities in other countries around the world, and least honoring of other methods available to support the patient's body in its recovery.(1)

Dr. Lerner suggests that nutritional therapies are soon to be honored medically for their contributions to the recovery of a patient from disease, due to the extensive amount of data being gathered which is pointing in that direction.

Recently, a new Office of Alternative Medicine in the National Institutes of Health has been established, which is beginning rigorous scientific investigations into the credibility of the many treatment options being offered to patients outside of standard medical treatment.(3) This is an exciting new step for Western medicine, with the potential of opening up new options for the medical community in treating patients.

It is important for the patient and family to be aware that in the middle of alternative treatment can be found charlatans, who have their eye on the patient's pocketbook, rather than their well-being. ACS has available guidelines available in a free pamphlet (#8249) to help the patient and family to sort out what it considers valid options and what to be cautious of. Call 1-800-ACS-2345 for more information.

   Sources: (1) *Choice In Cancer*, by Michael Lerner, Ph.D.; (2) "General Information on Questionable Methods of Cancer Treatment," American Cancer Society #8249; (3) "NCCS Experts on Complementary Therapies to Top Assembly," *Networker* 7(3), [National Coalition for Cancer Survivorship] Summer 1993.

NUTRITION

Nutrition does seem to impact in some ways the prevention, treatment, and cure of cancer, though there are yet many unanswered questions. The American Cancer Society lists ten significant nutritional factors to keep in mind with regard to cancer: five protective factors and five risk factors(8):

Protective Factors:
1) Eat more cabbage-family vegetables
2) Add more high-fiber foods
3) Choose foods with Vitamin A
4) Choose foods with Vitamin C
5) Control your weight

Risk Factors:
1) Trim fat from your diet
2) Subtract salt-cured, smoked, nitrite-cured foods
3) Stop cigarette smoking
4) Go easy on alcohol
5) Respect the sun's rays

In addition, excessive X-rays, estrogens, and work-related chemicals and fibers like asbestos are listed as potential risks.

NUTRITION DURING CANCER TREATMENT

"A good rule to follow is to eat a variety of different foods every day. No one food or group of foods contains all of the nutrients you need. A diet to keep your body strong will include daily servings from these food groups:"(3)
1) Fruits and Vegetables
2) Protein Foods
3) Grains
4) Dairy Foods

Healthful snacks, adding variety to the menu, eating frequently, and changing time, place, and surroundings of meals may boost the appetite. Try softer foods, such as milkshakes or bananas *if the mouth gets sore.* Your tastes may change, so be creative and try new foods! *For dry mouth,* choose foods that hold more moisture or stimulate more saliva, such as sweet or tart foods. *For nausea,* try foods such as toast and crackers, sherbet, pretzels, or ice chips, and avoid fat, greasy, or fried foods. *For diarrhea,* try foods high in protein and calories, but low in fiber, such as yogurt, rice or noodles, white bread, or fish. *For constipation,* drink plenty of liquids, eat high-fiber foods (such as whole grains), raw fresh vegetables, and get some exercise (such as walking). *For weight gain during chemotherapy treatment,* know that it is probably due to water gain. *It is not recommended that you go on a diet during cancer treatment.*(3) *(See* "Eating Hints," National Cancer Institute #91-2079, for more details.)

Beating Cancer with Nutrition

Several excellent books are currently available that address the significance of nutrition for the patient going through cancer treatment. Malnutrition, due to a number of factors, including "depression, inactivity, pain, digestion and other physical problems, internal obstruction and reactions to the drugs…"(6) can significantly impact the cancer patient. "The right nutritional choices can often prevent, control, and reverse some of the adverse side effects of chemotherapy. They can also help build and maintain general health and thus improve chances of successful treatment and recovery…[T]he malnourished or marginally-nourished patient experiences more drug side effects. As a result, the treatment is then generally refused or curtailed, which in turn may permit the cancer to progress."(6)

Isn't the IV (intravenous) nutrition sufficient for the patient going through cancer treatment? The IV liter (1000 cc) bag of 5 percent dextrose (D5W), which may be given the cancer patient at times during treatment for hydrating and certain drug deliveries, contains no more than 170 calories, which is not as many calories as one might receive from a small breakfast muffin. The IV is *not* intended to be the main source of nutrition over the long term.(7)

Dr. Patrick Quillan, in his book *Beating Cancer with Nutrition,* suggests that as high as 40 percent of cancer patients may die from malnutrition going through cancer treatment. Whether or not the reader finds these numbers believable, it is important for the patient to be aware that current literature regarding prevention and treatment of cancer patients is beginning to take seriously the nutritional component in the fight against cancer. Therefore it is highly recommended that a patient and/or loved one review one or more of these nutritional books so that the patient is aware of the choices that can be made for a healthy diet to support well-being and recovery while going through cancer treatment.

Sources: (1) *Beating Cancer with Nutrition,* by Patrick Quillin, Ph.D., R.D.; (2) "Diet, Nutrition and Cancer Prevention," *The Good News* [National Cancer Institute] #87-2878; (3) "Eating Hints," National Cancer Institute #91-2079; (4) "The Good News," National Cancer Institute #87-2878; (5) "Eating Smart," American Cancer Society; (6) *Nutrition for the Chemotherapy Patient,* by Janet L. Ramstack, Dr. P. H. and Ernest H. Rosenbaum, M.D.; (7) *Nutrition and the Cancer Patient,* by Jane Bradley and Susan Nass; (8) "Taking Control: Ten Steps to a Healthier Life and Reduced Cancer Risk," American Cancer Society; (9) "What You Need to Know About Cancer," National Cancer Institute #90-1566.

TREATMENT RESEARCH

There is extensive research going on world-wide to try to address the more than 100 forms of cancer, and the best methods of treatment and cure.

"From an extremely complex group of findings, we are busy simultaneously trying to understand the cause of cancer and also to treat it. Molecular biologists and biochemists are hard at work on the former task, and from their still incomplete findings, pharmacologists are working to come up with drugs that will save people's lives."(1)

Some of the most active areas of interest in research are immunotherapy, biological agents, and antibody therapy.

Immunotherapy attempts to increase the effectiveness of the body's natural ability to fight disease, the immune system, through a number of techniques—for example, stimulating killer T-cells by the stimulation of macrophages.

Biological Agents: Many attempts at using biological agents to fight disease have been made through the years. Currently, the use of biological response modifiers, which "have no direct antitumor effect, but are able to trigger or stimulate the immune system and so indirectly affect tumors," is being explored.(2) The following list, taken from Dollinger, Rosenbaum, and Cable's *Everyone's Guide to Cancer Therapy,* describes some of these agents, all of which are being actively researched:

- *Interferons* (IFN) are a type of cytokine with antitumor properties, which are effective in shrinking melanoma and kidney tumors of some patients.
- *Interleukins* (IL-1 through IL-11) increase the activity of lymphocytes, part of the body's armament against foreign agents.
- *Colony Stimulating Factors* (CSFs) increase the activity of the number of neutrophils and/or macrophages, which, for example, lessen the risk for infection, thus allowing patients to recover much more quickly from high-dose chemotherapy.

- *T-Cells* recognize tumor cells and help encourage their destruction, "by either making helper factors that stimulate the rest of the immune system or making killer factors that destroy tumor cells."(2)
- *Tumor vaccines* are used the same way as other vaccines, such as polio. They have been effective in about 25 percent of patients with melanoma and kidney cancers and have prolonged the life of patients with some other types of cancers.
- *Tumor Necrosis Factors* (TNFs) are proteins that can destroy tumor cells. They "occur naturally in the body in small numbers and can be produced in a laboratory by stimulating macrophages and lymphocytes."(2)

Antibody Therapy: Antibodies are proteins produced by B lymphocytes, which recognize foreign substances and have an attached marker; this marker is identified by cells of the immune system, which then attack and attempt to destroy the foreign substance, e.g., Monoclonal Antibodies (MAbs), which are produced in the laboratory with the goal of targeting specific foreign body substances, such as cancer cells.

Sources: (1) *Breast Cancer,* by Yashar Hirshaut, M.D., F.A.C.P., and Peter I. Pressman, M.D., F.A.C.S.; (2) *Everyone's Guide to Cancer Therapy,* by Malin Dollinger, M.D., Ernest H. Rosenbaum, M.D., and Greg Cable.

NETWORK OF SUPPORT

"Cancer can be utterly lonely.
No one should try to bear it alone."(8)

Sharing a diagnosis of cancer with family and loved ones, as openly as you, the patient, are able, helps to begin the process of building bridges of communication across the chasms of fear and loneliness that accompany this illness. *During doctor's visits, it is helpful to have someone accompany the patient if at all possible*—not only for personal support, but to assist in collecting and sorting out the medical information offered the patient. Due to the high stress experienced by the patient dealing with a cancer diagnosis, *being able to take in and/or remember all of the details given at a doctor's appointment is most difficult.* If someone supportive is present at these times, the information gathered is often more accurate and complete, making decisions easier for the patient.

Choosing the people with whom to share the diagnosis, and how, is important. If there are people, including children, that you feel should know but do not feel up to the task for some reason, asking a friend or loved one to handle it is quite appropriate. When children are informed, it needs to be done in a way that is appropriate to their age and emotional maturity.

Becoming aware of the kind of support system you prefer to have as you walk through breast cancer is a part of the experience. Beginning to move in a direction to help make it happen comes next. The awareness of what is needed evolves in its own time as one moves through the experience of cancer. Respecting your own unique way of processing all that is happening to you and your family, and honoring the time it takes to personally work it through, is important to your well-being. It will give you back some sense of control in your life, and will also help support the well-being of those around you, because you are more at ease with what you have decided.

Take the time you need to make the decisions necessary regarding breast cancer treatment. Get a second opinion if you feel it is warranted.

> "Breast cancer should be treated as soon as possible, but that does not mean within a day or two and it certainly doesn't mean that speed is more important than making sound decisions...Tell any doctor who may be urging great haste upon you that you'd rather go home now and that you'll call him tomorrow or the next day..."
>
> —Yashar Hirshaut, M.D., F.A.C.P. and Peter I. Pressman, M.D., F.A.C.S., *Breast Cancer: A Complete Guide.*

It is important for the patient and loved ones to become aware that there are hundreds of breast cancer organizations in existence today just for the purpose of being there for a person and their family who has just been given a diagnosis of cancer. Most have been created by survivors of breast cancer and others who have been touched by the overwhelming aspects of this disease and simply want to assist others through the hoops.

> *Honor your uniqueness, your individuality, in all of the choices to come. Trust yourself. Find out what you need to know, as an individual, to make your decisions and allow those next to you to do the same, including your children, respecting what each needs to know. Respect that it is your life, your body, and your decisions that will count. No one else has the right to make those for you. Be your own best support person first. Then engage with others.*

SHIFTING RELATIONSHIPS

Know that you may see many shifts of relationships in your life during the journey through breast cancer. This is normal, and there are reasons for it.

1) *There are death and dying issues* which all who choose to interface with a patient with breast cancer typically must face. With the high value given to being young and youthful in our culture, there seems to be an accompanying denial that we must all one day die. Because death is not a comfortable subject for many Americans, when a person is diagnosed with cancer, the experience, and sometimes the patient, becomes the real life symbol of "death."

It is not uncommon for a breast cancer patient to be approached on this issue: "How do you feel about dying?" a patient might be asked. How, indeed, do we *all* feel about dying, one might ask. In fact, in inter-facing with many breast cancer patients, the facing of the issue of her/his mortality is one of the most difficult, yet empowering aspects of the breast cancer experience. Appreciating each moment one lives is the spin-off; not taking any lovely thing for granted can be a dramatic shift of perspective.

However, some people connected to the person diagnosed may be too uncomfortable with the issue of death to handle it yet, or there may be other challenges in their lives to make dealing with the issue too energy consuming at the time, so they choose to distance themselves either for the duration, or for periods of time, so that they can have more time to adjust more comfortably to the reality.

2) *The experiences surrounding breast cancer are very intense.* For the patient, as well as those who choose to support the patient, being a part of this experience requires great flexibility, a high degree of caring, plus enormous patience, dedication, and endurance. ***Everyone, including the patient, needs "time out" from breast cancer.*** This can take many creative forms: camping, climbing, art, drumming, medita-tion, a weekend away. Like the 15-minute breaks recommended in the business world to improve productivity, delightful mental breaks taken when needed will energize both the patient and support people involved.

One spouse said it well: "The not knowing is the worst." *So many things are unknown in this arena, and staying with that is difficult.* The spouse or loved one may feel he or she is responsible for the patient getting breast cancer and feeling enormous guilt, which may stay with him (or her) for many years.

Known causes and curative treatments for breast cancer sit firmly in a gray area, though there is new hope, including treatment with more predictable results, particularly for early-stage breast cancers. Information comes out almost daily. What treatment would I be wise to choose? Will there be, or what kind of short-term or long-term side effects will there be from treatment? Will I have a husband/wife/ partner/loved one when this is done? What kinds of financial strain will accompany this disease? Who will take over the motherly duties in the family? How will I, the children, and my loved ones cope? What about job opportunities after breast cancer? Increased job stress for those who choose to support a patient? The list goes on, so *respecting the intensity of the experience and making plans to diffuse the tensions regularly will significantly help.* This can be done on an individual basis or with group support. Supporting the development of a raucous sense of humor (I call it "trench humor") also helps. *The most bizarre things with cancer can make you laugh.* Allow it to happen.

RESPECTING PERSONAL STYLES

To best support one's own personal style of needed support, *it is highly recommended that the patient and/or her loved ones make a solid connection to a local breast cancer information/social support system.* You will be glad you did. Then, when questions arise, you will have the information available you need to make the appropriate choices for you, and the necessary social and emotional support to help you all move more smoothly through the journey. Just knowing there is a person available as close as the phone who can answer, or help you get the answer, to any question that arises is worth the connection.

CANCER SUPPORT CENTERS

Cancer information and support centers are most often a part of, or connected to the services of an accredited hospital or medical clinic, though there are independent centers available, as well. *To locate a center near you, call the American Cancer Society, 1-800-ACS-2345.*

Each cancer information and support center may vary in the specific services offered patients, depending on their philosophy, staff available, the population they are serving, what type of medical, financial, and community support they have in place, and what kind of facility they have available.

The primary services usually offered through a cancer information and support center include:

1) *Informational Support* for the cancer patient and their loved ones: on-going, up-to-date information pertinent to the patient's specific needs, and the needs of her/his loved ones in the form of printed, visual, and audio materials, plus information on where they can connect in the community for other resources available to them.

2) *Classes* to educate and directly address specific needs of the patients and loved ones related to the disease in a group format.

3) *Social-Emotional Support* offered in the form of support groups, oncology social workers, and/or volunteers for the cancer patient and loved ones.

The center may also involve themselves quite extensively in *Community Education*, such as classes offered in the community on how to do breast self-exams, or the importance of mammograms. The center may also invite those from the community to be a part of classes, or presentations held at the medical facility with a variety of presenters, such as health care personnel, medical specialists, or those with expertise in tai chi, nutrition, or relaxation techniques.

The advantage of connecting to a cancer information and support center is that the patient and family can be in ongoing contact with people who are current with treatment and other issues connected to breast cancer and whose sole purpose is to give support to cancer patients in any way they can. Such a group will probably be aware of the financial, legal, and political issues surrounding this arena. They are also typically in touch with a broader state and national network of breast cancer support groups, which can be of enormous benefit.

Sources: (1) Deborah Shiro, Program Manager, Detection, Washington Division, American Cancer Society; (2) Judith Jones, Cancer Education Specialist, Kirkland, WA.

"The diagnosis of cancer usually hits most of us with a wave of shock, of fright, of denial. Each person needs a different length of time to pull himself or herself together to deal with the reality of cancer."(8)

WHOM SHOULD I TELL?

Choose to tell the people you feel up to telling. If you want others to know whom you don't feel up to telling, allow others close to you to assist you in that task. *If there are children, be open to them, but sensitive to their age and emotional maturity, in addition to their personal choices* of what they want to know when. Children are much more aware than we give them credit for, and will imagine worse things than if we are simply honest with them. They have a remarkable capacity for handling difficult circumstances if they are given the facts openly to deal with.

"As you ponder whether you can share the diagnosis of cancer with others, it might help to remember...[that]...in telling the people you love... you have cancer, you give them the opportunity to express their feelings, to voice their fears and hopes and to offer their hand in support. Then, each can give and take strength as they are able."(8)

ASKING FOR HELP

Others will want to help you, but many times will just not know what to do. The more specific you can be about the help you need, the better, according to Judy Jones, Cancer Information Specialist. Keep a list of the things that you feel need to be done, and when someone asks, let them know, and perhaps choose one from the list of things you have to do that might fit into their life at that time. They will thank you, and you will get something necessary accomplished, which will help you both.

SUGGESTION: *On your list, put in some fun things, like putting flowers in a vase, reading a story to you and/or your children, renting a movie, or taking you for a walk on the beach. You will be glad you did.*

INDIVIDUAL OR GROUP COUNSELING

Consider counseling, either individual or group, if you think it might be helpful. Some hospitals offer such counseling as a part of standard care while you are in the hospital; others have outpatient counseling.(8) If it is not available through the local hospital, contact the American Cancer Society for information regarding the availability of cancer volunteers or therapists qualified in your community to counsel cancer patients. *Group support for breast cancer patients is often available free of charge in breast cancer support groups, or may also be available through a local therapist at a cost.*

SPIRITUAL HELP

For many women, spiritual support through their local church, synagogue, or spiritual support group is a great help during breast cancer. This can take on many cultural flavors, as well. Discovering what really works to support one's individual journey becomes one of the "jewels" a breast cancer patient picks up along the way and does not have to relinquish when it is over.

SEX AND BREAST CANCER

Sexuality is "one of the most sensitive and intimate aspects of a relationship...[and] is vulnerable to the ravages of serious illness and its treatment."(1)

According to Dr. David Spiegel, a pioneer in cancer support treatment for women with breast cancer, sexual problems can have a number of origins:

1) *The damage caused by an illness may limit sexual abilities.* For the woman with breast cancer, this might be seen in the loss of a breast, or discomfort from the side effects from cancer treatment.

2) *Sexual difficulties may result from the general loss of energy* that comes with being sick: of feeling sick, tired, or frightened. It takes a lot of energy to deal with having breast cancer.

3) *Disfigurement, weight loss, or weakness may leave you feeling undesirable,* even if you experience desire.

Dr. Spiegel suggests that you find ways of being open about any concerns you have to your sexual partner, and that you allow your partner to do the same, so that sensitive bridges of communication can be rebuilt to support a renewed intimate sexual relationship. Some people simply lose their sexual interest for a while, and eventually reconnect without too much adjustment. Others take more time and more commitment to deal with the changes that have occurred.

"Intimacy is the ultimate act of trust and acceptance, which means that in those first few intimate encounters, many other emotions may be intermingled with the passion as the woman begins to let down her guard and feel not only the good feelings of passion but the variety of other emotions connected to what has happened to her."(4)

Try to keep an open mind about ways to feel sexual pleasure as you work through the new adjustments. "These times can be a chance to learn new ways to give and receive sexual pleasure."(2) Know that cancer is not contagious: it is not given or "caught" from others.

SUGGESTION: *If vaginal dryness is a problem, or there is vaginal tenderness due to chemotherapy treatment, there are vaginal lubricants which may help. Common brands include Lubrin, Condom Mate suppositories, K-Y Jelly, Ortho Personal Lubricant, Surgilube, Today Personal Lubricant, and Astroglide.*

Sources: (1) *Living Beyond Limits*, by Dr. David Spiegel; (2) *Sexuality and Cancer: For the Woman Who Has Cancer and Her Partner.* American Cancer Society #4657-PS, 1988; (3) *Sexuality and Cancer: For the Man Who Has Cancer and His Partner.* American Cancer Society #4658-PS, 1988; (4) *The Breast Cancer Companion,* by Kathy LaTour.

SUPPORT GROUP OR NO SUPPORT GROUP?

Breast cancer support groups have been shown by Stanford University Psychiatrist Dr. David Spiegel to increase the survival of women with advanced breast cancer by an average of twice as long, giving medical credibility to the concept that *social and emotional support has a marked physical impact on the life of women with breast cancer.*(5) There is not yet data available for women with early-staged breast cancer. One of the additional benefits spoken to repeatedly by women I have interviewed is that, due to the still-unresolved medical issues surrounding breast cancer, a breast cancer support group offers them a rich pool of experiential knowledge available through other breast cancer survivors, which helps them sort out the enormous amount of medical information available, from which significant decisions need to be made.

However, according to Elaine Lachlan, Social Oncologist at Wellness Works (Kirkland, WA), *a breast cancer group does not work for everybody.* Some women prefer to process it on their own, within their own network of support already in place. Some women come for a time, and then do not return, or they may choose to return at a later date, due to recurrence, or, perhaps, just a felt need to be a part of the group, or reconnect to old friends. It is a very individual choice that needs to be respected for what it is. No one should feel forced to go to a support group.

CULTURAL STYLES

A patient support system needs to honor the *unique personal,* as well as cultural, processing styles. Each individual patient needs to feel supported in selecting her own pathway through this journey. No two individuals go through it exactly alike. Not every woman feels comfortable sharing personal things in a group setting, due to a number of important factors, nor is there cultural support for some styles. Some cultures support more of a group process—others, a more individual one. Therefore, when offering services to an individual patient, these unique preferences need to be taken into consideration.

American Indian

There are many different American Indian tribes in the United States; therefore a wide cultural diversity is represented. Still, there are a number of cultural patterns which tend to be present in many more traditional American Indian tribes that can impact the way an Indian woman with breast cancer processes her journey.

In an interview with Dr. June Strickland, who has done extensive work with Indian populations and cancer, and who is herself an American Indian, the following patterns were identified. In many Indian communities the culture is a *matriarchal community*. This means, among many other things, that *women are given high regard and status in the significant decision-making of a tribe.* Also, great value is given to *attentive listening skills*, with *few words spoken*—and only if something significant can be added in a group conversation. *A manner of quiet speaking* is highly valued.

These characteristics play out significantly in an American Indian woman's interaction with the American medical community, which is typically patriarchal, with great value given to assertive, ready speech. If a medical doctor takes on an air of male superiority, offering little respect for the Indian woman who listens carefully, and speaks softly when she does speak, the result is viewed as disrespectful and distasteful by the American Indian woman, out of respect for herself and the things she values highly in her cultural context. She will typically not choose to return to such a doctor. The doctor may view her as non-assertive from his cultural perspective.

If breast cancer comes to an American Indian woman, she may choose *walks alone in nature, ceremony, reaching out to a tribal elder or to a medicine person to process the experience personally in a way that respects her cultural orientation.* Individuals of a tribe are taught from a very young age to work out their own problems, and those with more life experience and wisdom in the tribe are traditionally available to the tribal member for help. It is considered undesirable, and disrespectful of the individual, to force unsolicited help on one who is working through a difficult time. American Indian women may not feel comfortable participating in non-Indian breast cancer support groups.

— June Strickland, Ph.D. (Dr. Strickland has had extensive public health experience, including over 10 years in cancer outreach with American Indian populations.)

Asian

For the Asian woman (which includes *many diverse Asian cultures*), the American medical system typically offers a set of different challenges. *Highly modest,* an Asian woman might be much more reluctant than a Caucasian or African-American woman to disrobe for full examination in front of medical personnel. *Culturally patriarchal,* there is usually a *well-defined familial structure for processing matters of familial importance, with the male point of view traditionally holding the most value.*

In terms of personal processing, such a diagnosis as breast cancer would typically be considered something *not to be discussed in public,* since *public exposure of personal feelings is considered ill-mannered and undesirable.* In some Asian cultures, serious illness religiously might represent *bad karma* happening because of something she or someone in her family did in another lifetime. Publicly, then, it might represent a source of *public shame* for her and her family.

I am aware of several Japanese women where even the closest friends or family of a breast cancer patient are not aware of any details of her illness, and in another case, where the mother of a young Chinese woman with breast cancer has refused to speak with her daughter in any way regarding the illness. The young Chinese woman, married to a Caucasian, has chosen to be very open publicly with her illness, a source of great embarrassment to her mother.

An Asian woman's choice of *alternative medical support* might include the practice of *tai chi* and/or *a selection of Chinese herbal medicines* (both quite commonly used outside Asian cultures). She may also offer *prayers and offerings to her ancestors.* The use of *"coin rubbing"* (the practice of repeatedly rubbing the skin with the edge of a coin, or *"cupping"* (the practice of putting a small lit candle on the skin, and placing a cup or small bowl over it, which creates a suction), might be used in some Chinese cultures to help the patient get rid of the illness. The medical community, to be most effective in attempting to support an Asian woman's journey through breast cancer, needs to respect the cultural context in which she lives.

— Elaine Dao, A.R.N.P., Director of Nursing Services, Kinon Nursing Home (Seattle, WA).

African-American

The African-American woman's experience may well involve an added layer of *unspoken racial prejudice for being black in a predominately white medical community,* which may compromise the care offered her by the medical community. According to Georgiana Arnold, Health Care Professional, Project Director of the W.K. Kellogg Community-Based Public Health Initiative, this *compromised health care is often an unconscious act by health care professionals.* This added challenge for African-American women was first pointed out to me by an African-American woman, a public school principal who battled with not only breast cancer, but lupus at the same time. She spoke of the medical community's lack of respect for her time with regard to pre-scheduled treatment appointments as compared to her business obligations, and to the life and death issues involving two other members of her family—one male and one female adult—located in the south where, in her view, medical decisions were at times overlaid with the biased view that their lives as blacks were not considered to hold as much value as a white person with the same illness, resulting in medical care that was significantly compromised. She was outraged at what her family members had to deal with and the degree of time and effort necessary to get some of the issues resolved.

Arnold states: "Many African-American women have *formal and informal support systems comprised of other African-American women.* These women frequently (but not always) turn to these supportive *'sister friends'* to share information about their health." She goes on to say that the African-American woman's network of support may also include "a *large extended family composed of blood relatives and close friends who have demonstrated their love, loyalty, and reliability through the years... African-American men can also be a crucial part of the support/recovery process* for their wives, lovers, mothers, sisters, and friends."

In some communities, depending on the black woman's culture, socioeconomic and educational background, the use of *herbs and other non-allopathic medicines* (those other than standard medical treatment) might be used by the African-American woman *combined with the standard medical treatment.* Most black women make use of the standard treatment offered by the medical community, though for many there remains a deep-seated distrust of the medical system, especially of white male physicians. This distrust, according to Arnold, may cause them to delay seeking medical care. African-American women particularly appreciate the support of committed, sensitive African-American health care providers.

A diagnosis of breast cancer may not be readily accepted among black women, states Arnold, *since it is seen more typically as a white woman's disease.* In addition, *many African-Americans equate a diagnosis of cancer with death, or an "act of God," and so may not actively engage in preventive and/or health screening behaviors.*

Interfacing on a regular basis may also be complicated for the black woman, due to so many *economic and childcare responsibilities,* which encourage them "to ignore their health until they experience significant symptoms for a long period of time."(Arnold) So, even though, according to the American Cancer Society, there are fewer black women who are diagnosed with breast cancer, when they are diagnosed, it is typically found in a more advanced stage and with more serious consequences.

> "In addition to racial and gender bias, African-American women face a medical system that favors and rewards female patients who are: compliant (don't disagree too often or ask too many questions); exhibit a communication style (accent, intonation and inflection) that closely resembles that of the staff; and appear to resemble the socioeconomic background of the health care practitioners."
>
> — Georgiana Arnold, Health Care Professional, Project Director of the W.K. Kellogg Community-Based Public Health Initiative, Seattle, WA

Hispanic

The Hispanic woman, along with some Asian cultures, may come into the experience of breast cancer with a *language barrier.* This holds great significance for a woman seeking to understand the choices she might have available in the American medical system. *Accurate information and choices may not always be communicated* to the monolingual-Spanish- or limited-English-speaking patient, as medical staff have often depended on untrained and nonprofessional individuals such as housekeepers or others to act as the legal medical "interpreter" between the doctor and the patient in a medical context.

The Hispanic patient often needs a medical advocate to speak on her/his behalf and to act as interpreter and guide through the American medical system, with which the patient is unfamiliar. Lack of understanding of the Hispanic culture and language by the vast majority of those providing care to cancer patients is of great concern for Hispanic health care givers. For example, it is not unusual for the Hispanic patient to *give great deference to the doctor,* to the point that questions may not be asked, because the doctor's time is given such great value. *Courtesy is considered of great importance culturally,* so it will be evidenced in the interaction with medical personnel, sometimes at the expense of the needs of the patient.

When a Hispanic woman comes to see a doctor, it is not unusual to see a number of family members accompanying her. There is a *strong traditional family network of support,* which also functions as a *decision-making group* where matters of concern that affect the family are typically discussed and decided upon, not unlike some Asian cultures. The Hispanic male spouse, functioning in a *patriarchal culture,* might be quite uncomfortable having another male, even though he may be a medical doctor, view his wife's breast for examination, so *the woman may not get the support necessary to see the doctor.*

— Carolina Lucero, Home Care Division Director,
SEA MAR Community Health Centers, Seattle, WA

One breast cancer surgeon shared two instances in his practice—one Asian, and one Arabian—where *the male spouse made the decision for breast cancer treatment regarding the woman's health. The woman had no say.* Another breast cancer surgeon shared the fact that *in some Caucasian marriages in his practice, the woman defers to the husband in breast cancer treatment choices*, though the surgeon consciously works to interface primarily with the woman to respect her medical choices.

Cultural bias is a very significant issue for **lesbian women** with breast cancer, who must go through the medical community for medical support. *(See* Lesbians and Breast Cancer.) They *typically do not interface on a regular basis with the medical community due to cultural bias and economic challenges.*

What does all this multi-cultural information mean? It seems to indicate that there are, indeed, multi-cultural medical issues that need to be much more thoroughly identified. Then, we need to address them directly when attempting to offering medical services to such a widely diverse cultural base as is found in the United States. These few observations from just a small group of individuals, though they represent many years of broad experience both personally and professionally, suggest we have only scratched the surface. There must be much more information available from the many additional cultures we represent as a country, which may prove to be quite profound when identified. The individual patients and health care specialists who have shared openly their keen observations of cultural diversity as represented in patients they deal with in our medical system, pose a number of significant questions that beg to be answered. *Is the medical community aware of the implications of cultural diversity represented in a medical context across the United States? Is the medical community as a whole being trained adequately to deal effectively with cultural diversity as it plays out in medical services offered for the American population? Is the American woman who is a member of a minority culture at increased risk because of her cultural and/or economic orientation? If so, what can be done about it?*

CONCLUSION: *There appear to be multi-cultural and minority cultural elements that need to be addressed with respect to medical care and breast cancer, so that women with this disease can be ultimately more individually respected as they traverse the difficult road to recovery. Just how this piece may play out for women in our medical system is yet to be fully understood.*

THE PATIENT-DOCTOR RELATIONSHIP

Becoming a partner in the relationship with your doctor is very important. It is your life and well-being at stake. You have employed this person—a doctor—and other medical personnel to assist you in a recovery process, and they have agreed to do what they can. *There are a number of things you and your support people can do to encourage a good partnership with the medical staff.* The following list of ideas have been developed from Dr. David Spiegel's support groups in his book, *Living Beyond Limits.*

1) *Humanize your relationship with your physician.* Remember you are both just people doing a job together at a select point in time.
2) *Write down your questions.* Think through what you feel is important to relay to your doctor in the time you have together. It is the most effective use of your appointment time and also respects his time restraints.
3) *Announce at the beginning of the interview that you have questions.*

Judith Jones, Director of Wellness Works through the Evergreen Cancer Center (Kirkland, WA), addresses a significant issue with regard to doctor choices for the patient. She indicates that, when possible, a patient needs to be supported in choosing a doctor that fits her personality style, in addition to the matter of professional credibility.

Some patients, she points out, prefer to have the best medical team technically available, and will give up a little on the doctor's "bedside manner," the doctor's personal style of communicating with the patient.

Other patients prefer a more supportive "bedside manner," to extensive medical credits and technical ability.

Some patients, she observes, want to know all of the medical information possible before making a decision, and some prefer to handle less, some as little as possible. It is in the best interest of the patient who prefers more information to connect to a doctor whose philosophy and personal style support a more active patient interaction. And, for the woman who would prefer not to know all the details, that her choice of doctor(s) reflects someone who is able to respect her orientation to the medical community.

The perfect choice for one patient, therefore, may not be the right choice for the next patient. Being aware of this issue could save a patient—and the medical team—much grief.

INFORMATION SUPPORT:
Call the National Cancer Institute at 1-800-4-CANCER,
the American Cancer Society at 1-800-ACS-2345,
or Commonweal (Information available on alternative treatments)
(415) 868-0790.
Also, see the Bibliography at the end of this volume.

PATIENT SUPPORT:

CanSurmount: A program where a newly diagnosed cancer patient is matched according to the type of cancer, age, and sex with a recovered patient, for a visitation. *Call the American Cancer Society for more details.*

Reach to Recovery: A program where a breast cancer patient still in the hospital is visited by a breast cancer survivor who brings a kit of useful items to help support her recovery, and who describes a set of specific exercises to regain the physical range of motion in her arm and chest on the affected side. *Call the American Cancer Society if you would like to be contacted.*

The following are a few *regional cancer support groups* available to the public. To find a more complete listing, contact the American Cancer Society at 1-800-ACS-2345.

Cancer Care: New York, NY (212) 302-2400.

Commonweal: Bolinas, CA (914) 967-6080.

Exceptional Cancer Patients New Haven, CT (203) 865-8392;

The Wellness Community: Santa Monica, CA
(310) 453-2200

Sources: 1) *Cancer as a Turning Point,* by Lawrence LeShan, M.D.; 2) "Living with Cancer," *Coping,* May/June 1993; 3) *From Victim to Victor, The Wellness Community Guide to Fighting for Recovery for Cancer Patients and Their Families,* by Harold H. Benjamin, M.D.; 4) *I Can Cope,* By Judi Johnson and Linda Klein; 5) *Living Beyond Limits,* by David Spiegel, M.D.; 6) *Triumph: Getting Back to Normal When You Have Cancer,* by Marion Morra and Eve Potts; 7) Elaine

Lachlan, Social Oncologist, and 8) Judith Jones, Cancer Information Specialist, Wellness Works, Evergreen Cancer Center, Kirkland, WA.

PAIN

> "Patients with cancer often fear the pain associated with their diagnosis more than the diagnosis itself. While not all cancer patients experience pain, those who do have a right to pain relief."
>
> — "Pain Service," Swedish Tumor Institute, Swedish Medical Center, Seattle, WA

Not all breast cancer patients have physical pain. Early cancers hardly ever give patients a pain challenge, and "even more advanced cancers do not always have pain."(4) If pain does occur, there are current pain guidelines available for medical personnel, and the patient, for optimum control.(1,2) Pain *"can almost always...be relieved or controlled"*(4) *when handled by knowledgeable medical staff.*

Pain needs to be personally and medically respected since it can affect the patient in many ways.

"[Pain] can keep you from being active, from sleeping well, from enjoying family and friends, and from eating. Pain can also make you feel afraid or depressed."(2) It may also cause worry or concern for the patient's loved ones.

A couple of facts regarding **medical pain control:** (1) *Pain needs to be managed consistently, with doses of pain medication given regularly* to be most effective, rather than waiting until it peaks with intensity. The reason for regular doses is that handling pain only when it peaks does not work well: pain medicines have a much more difficult time controlling the pain when it is in "full bloom" than when the pain is handled regularly while it is yet of small-to-moderate intensity.(2) *"Getting hooked" or "addicted" to pain medicines rarely happens,* although it is frequently a fear of both patient and medical staff.

There may be **other medical pain solutions:** *radiation therapy* to reduce the spread of or pressure caused by the cancer; sometimes a *nerve block* is used when nothing else has worked.

There are also **nonmedical techniques** available that can help with pain. They usually have few to zero side effects, and can be combined with the medical techniques. It is currently not unusual to have someone trained on staff or connected to the hospital who is available to teach one or more of the following techniques to patients: *relaxation, imagery, meditation, prayer,* or *distraction by music, humor, art.* An infinite variety of personal choices can be made to connect to supportive, pleasurable outlets that can distract the mind/body for periods of time from the intensity of pain sensations being experienced by the patient.(3)

NOTE: *If you are not getting sufficient medical support for your pain, it may be that the medical personnel you are working with are not specially trained in pain control. You may call for a pain specialist from the hospice connected to one of the hospitals in your area for information about how to be better supported. Managing pain is typically one of their specialties.*

Call the American Cancer Society 1-800-ACS-2345
for information about local hospices in your area,
as well as more specific information regarding pain management.

Sources: (1) *Clinical Practice Guideline on Management of Cancer Pain,* by AHCPR (Agency for Health Care Policy and Research), 1994. Copy available by calling 1-800-4-CANCER); (2) *Managing Cancer Pain,* Consumer Version, Clinical Practice Guideline, #9, U.S. Department of Health and Human Services, 1994; (3) *Quantum Healing,* by Deepak Chopra, M.D.; (4) *Questions and Answers About Pain Control: A Guide for People with Cancer and Their Families,* American Cancer Society and National Cancer Institute. (Call 1-800-4-CANCER for a copy).

LESBIANS AND BREAST CANCER

Incidence: Lesbian women are thought to have two to three times the risk for breast cancer as women in the general population, according to data taken from several studies that included about 5,000 participants.(Susan Haynes, Epidemiologist at the National Cancer Institute, 2, 6) *Much more research is needed to more clearly understand the significant issues for lesbian women.*

Risk Factors are the same as for women of the general population. However, because some risk factors for all women are more common among lesbians, it does seem to indicate that lesbian women as a whole may be more at risk.

1) *Being a woman.*
2) *Aging.*
3) *No birth of a child.* Eighty-four percent of lesbian women who participated in a recent survey (1983-88) by the National Lesbian and Gay Health Care Foundation had no children.(2)
4) *Increased body fat.* Thirty-four percent of lesbian women compared to 28 percent of all women in US over 55 have increased body fat.(2)
5) *Alcohol consumption.* At least some lesbian women, according to a federally funded study in Kentucky, drink more than the average American woman.(2)
6) *Fewer routine medical exams.* Lesbian women are less likely to have regular medical exams because: a) *Experiences of cultural bias against, or discomfort with their sexual orientation in a medical context, during previous medical exams.* Thirty-four percent of lesbian women in a recent survey involving 2,000 participants did not have a regular Ob/Gyn for female exams.(4) b) Lesbians fear *the quality of their health care may be compromised due to their sexual orientation.* Evidence suggests this fear may be well-founded.(1) Thus, when a lesbian woman does go for help, the breast cancer is typically more advanced.(3)

"A woman who is battling cancer is generally not a woman who has the energy or patience to start educating her doctor about (being) lesbian. Yet she cannot afford to ignore incorrect assumptions that may affect her doctor's attitude or her plan of treatment."(1)

Since a lesbian partner has no legal standing in the medical community, complications arise repeatedly in hospital and medical care settings. "Many hospitals won't let a sick woman's partner into the intensive care unit because she is not considered immediate family."(1) Or, the patient's family's discomfort with the lesbian relationship may make it very difficult for the partner to be part of the patient's ongoing support system.

There are no risk factors that are lesbian-specific, but some of the risk factors that are listed for the general population of women may occur more frequently [among lesbians]. (Fran Visco, President of the National Breast Cancer Coalition, 2)

"It's almost a moot point whether lesbians are at a greater risk than other women. [Breast cancer] is an epidemic."
— Susan Love, M.D., *Dr. Susan Love's Breast Book.*
[*Love is involved in two efforts to study lesbian breast cancer.(2)*]

SUGGESTION: *It is advisable for all patients, both lesbian women and other breast cancer patients, to take time to give a complete list to the medical doctor(s) in charge of the people who are to be considered "family members" in terms of shared information, or being present at the time of any medical consultations. This is important because of the legalities surrounding the "privacy" issues that medical personnel are required to respect. For instance, unless a patient gives the doctor the okay, no medical information can be shared with other members of the family, including the spouse or partner. It causes significant complications for the medical community when this issue is not taken care of at the start of treatment.*

Taking care of this does not, however, protect the patient from cultural bias of being lesbian, or stop other family members from trying to block information from and participation with those they do not wish to be a part of the patient's "family" network, even though legally, the patient, if of legal age, has the right to choose who is privy to his/her medical information.

Caitlin Ryan, a social worker and chief of the AIDS office of the District of Columbia, directed the National Lesbian Health Care survey in 1985. Her findings: of almost 2,000 women surveyed, 70 percent had not given birth, 21 percent over 50 were heavy drinkers, and 34 percent referred to weight problems. Suzanne G. Haynes, epidemiologist with the National Cancer Institute, used this data as the basis to calculate lesbians' breast cancer risk factors. She found that lesbian women have a "two- to three-fold" higher risk factor than other women. Be aware that all women have less of a risk factor when they are young, and that it increases as they age. This increase with age remains true for lesbian women, as well.

Sources: (1) *Bringing It Home,* by Lynn Kanter, 1993; (2) *Lesbians and Breast Cancer,* by Marsha Gessen. *The Advocate,* 1993; (3) Liz Ilg, Seattle Lesbian Cancer Project, Seattle WA; (4) Marion Lynch, M.D., Fellow in Cancer Prevention, Fred Hutchinson Cancer Research Center, Seattle, WA; (5) *The Politics of Breast Cancer: Are Lesbians a High-Risk Group for Breast Cancer?* by Kate Rounds, *Ms.* May/June 1993; (6) "Lesbians and Breast Cancer," National Cancer Institute, February 9, 1993.

Community Resources for Lesbian Women : (1) National Coalition of Feminist and Lesbian Cancer Projects, P.O. Box 90437, Washington, DC 20090. Phone: 202-332-5536. [*Dedicated to the empowerment of grassroots women's cancer groups, and committed to"creating an organization through which feminist and lesbian cancer projects can work for changes on a national level."*] (2) Seattle Lesbian Cancer Project, 2732 N.E. 54th St. Seattle, WA 98105. Phone: 206-522-0199 [*A grassroots feminist organization dedicated to providing access to lesbians sensitive health care services for lesbians living with cancer and their families. Also has available a list of other organizations supportive of lesbian issues.*]

MALE BREAST CANCER

For the most up-to-date information on male breast cancer, call 1-800-4-CANCER (National Cancer Institute) or 1-800-ACS-2345 (American Cancer Society)

Incidence: Breast cancer is rare in men. According to the American Cancer Society, of 183,000 new breast cancer cases expected in 1994, only 1,000 of these are expected to be men. Of those, 46,000 women and 300 men are expected to die of the disease. *Breast cancer tends to occur in middle aged, or elderly men and seems to occur more in men with gynecomastia (enlarged male breasts).*

Risk Factors: Rarely, families may have multiple cases of male breast cancer. *Gynecomastia* (enlargement of the male breast) predisposes men to the disease.(2) There is some evidence to suggest that male breast cancer appears to be *associated with Klinefelter's syndrome* (a genetic disease associated with gynecomastia [enlargement of the male breast]). (2) Men with *hyperestrogenism* (increased levels of estrogen) are at higher risk.(2)

Symptoms: Breast lumps, usually firm and painless, most typically located just below the nipple or areola. Abnormality of the nipple: retracted nipple, crusting or discharge from the nipple and ulceration. Rather uncommon (10 percent), but when present, highly symptomatic.(3)

Often presents as a localized disease in about 44 percent of cases, and 45 percent as a regional disease.(2)

Usually found at a more advanced stage of disease than females due to the fact that males do not consider breast cancer a possible male disease, so they do not typically follow discovery with a doctor's exam.

TYPES OF TUMORS

Resembles breast cancer in women, with the exception that lobular carcinoma is seldom seen.(2) Most commonly found tumors are: *infiltrating ductal carcinoma*, 85 percent(3), *medullary carcinoma* and *papillary carcinoma*, both about 5 percent(3), *tubular carcinoma, adenocystic carcinoma,* and *carcinosarcoma.*

FACTORS USED FOR DIAGNOSIS

Physical examination with complete medical history, blood studies, and X-ray (typically a mammogram).(2)

Biopsy: Taken by needle aspiration or by standard excisional/ incisional biopsy. (This test is essential for confirming the diagnosis.) Hormone receptor test offers valuable treatment and prognostic information.

Staging: Same system used as for females, with the observation that men usually are diagnosed at a more advanced stage. *(See* Staging of Breast Cancer)

Prognosis: Depends on how advanced the disease is at the time of diagnosis, patient's medical condition, the extent of the tumor, and patient's response to treatment.(2) Localized Disease: 97 percent survival rate at 5 years. Non-Regional Disease: 77 percent survival rate at five years.

Treatment: **Standard approach:** *radical mastectomy,* due to closeness of tumors to pectoralis major muscle and to the more advanced stage breast cancer found in males.(5)

Modified radical mastectomy is now being used in earlier stages of the disease (smaller tumors, less cancer involvement).(5)

Also, a portion of the pectoralis major muscle beneath the tumor may be surgically removed to create a clear margin of safety.

Radiation therapy: may be used alone in early stages of breast cancer, postoperatively following a mastectomy, or in advanced cancer to relieve symptoms.(5)

Dr. Paul R. Reich suggests that some patients benefit from the removal of the testicles to decrease the production of androgen, which figures in the growth of the tumor. Also, large doses of estrogen, female hormones, may be used to help relieve symptoms.(6)

Adjuvant Chemotherapy: Used frequently in patients with Stage II or above breast cancer. Similar to treatment for women.(3)

Adjuvant Hormone Therapy: Tamoxifen most typically used for Stage II or above breast cancer. Similar to treatment for women.(3)

LONG-TERM EFFECTS

Long-term effects for male breast cancer patients may include a decreased function of shoulder, arm edema, and stiffness and pain in the radiated area, or surgical part of the chest wall. There may also be psychological after-effects.(2)

Additional Comments:

Male breast cancer is too uncommon to allow randomized clinical trials of systemic therapy, so most decisions are based on research for women.

- *Regular mammograms are not recommended for males* due to the small number of men who contact the disease. However, men with gynecomastia may be wise to practice breast self examinations.
- Doctors may not consider breast cancer as a strong possibility for a breast lump compared to a woman, so *a male may need to be more aggressive in the medical community to get an accurate diagnosis.*
- *Men need to be aware that breast cancer is not just a woman's disease.*

Sources: (1) "Breast Cancer Strikes 1,000 Men Annually," by Heidi Nolte Brown. *Journal American* [Bellevue, WA], July 19, 1993; (2) "Cancer of the Male Breast: Diagnosis," American Cancer Society #407172; (3) "Male Breast Cancer," by Christopher J. Williams, and Roger B. Buchanan. *Textbook of Uncommon Cancer,* John Wiley & Sons, 1991, pp.827-835; (4) "Male Breast Cancer," by David W. Kinne, M.D., and Thomas B. Hakes. *Breast Diseases:* J. B. Lippincott & Company, 1991, pp.782-790; (5) "Management of Male Breast Cancer," by David W. Kinne, M.D. *Oncology,* 5(2): 45-48, March 1991; (6) *The Facts About Chemotherapy,* by Paul R. Reich, M.D. 1991.

"This cancer is like an obnoxious child that just won't mind. It just keeps coming back...I'm young, and have a lot of living to do still. I don't want to die."

— Tara Havemeyer, breast cancer warrior

BREAST CANCER RECURRENCE

"The risks of recurrence of breast cancer have gone way down in recent years. Unfortunately, even with the best treatment and the most meticulous follow-up care, cancer may recur."(3)

It isn't fair, to have gone through cancer treatment before in order to put it behind you, and here it is back. Many women with breast cancer who find themselves in these shoes have shared with me how much more difficult it is the second time. Can I do this again? Is it worth the effort? Is there any treatment left that will make a difference?

Yes, there is treatment available that can be called up to reign in the illness and permit a woman with recurrence to live a normal life, often for many years. And, yes, there are breast cancer patients that put together a combined treatment program of their choice that somehow puts breast cancer away from them forever. "What is required—from both the patient and the physician—is a determined effort, a forceful attack."(3) Where the cancer has recurred, either local (in the same area as before), or distant (cancer that has metastasized, or spread to another location in the body) determines to a large degree the treatment choices made. Surgery, chemotherapy, radiation, and hormone therapy may be used for treatment. "It may come back in the breast, in the soft tissues of the chest (the chest wall), or in another part of the body," according to the National Cancer Institute. ("Breast Cancer," *PDQ Information for Patients,* 10/31/94.

Much research is being addressed in the direction of advanced cancer treatment. *You may want to be a part of a clinical study that tries out a new treatment.* Discuss thoroughly with your doctor the options available to you. Get a second opinion if you desire. Call NCI at 1-800-4-CANCER for the latest information on your type of recurrence, and any ongoing clinical studies available for patients. DO carefully consider the choice of action you take. Then, call ACS at 1-800-ACS-2345 to see what kind of support systems are available for you and your family to help you work through this time. It is your body, and your life, after all.

Sources: (1) "Advanced Cancer," National Cancer Institute #93-856; (2) *Beating Cancer with Nutrition,* by Dr. Patrick Quillin; (3) *Breast Cancer,* Yahsar Hirshaut, M.D., F.A.C.P. and Peter I. Pressman, M.D., F.A.C.S.; (4) *Cancer as a Turning Point,* by Lawrence Leshan, Ph.D.; (5) *From Victim to Victor,* by Harold H. Benjamin, Ph.D.; (6) *I Can Cope,* by Judi Johnson, and Linda Klein; (7) *The Cancer Conqueror,* by Greg Anderson; (8) "When Cancer Recurs," National Cancer Institute #87-2709.

INSURANCE

"You can't be fired for being sick. Your health insurance can't be terminated if you get cancer, as long as you're able to do your job. The information you or your doctor provides in connection with an insurance claim is confidential. If you do leave your job, you are entitled to coverage at a group rate for a period of time until you can make other arrangements."(1)

All of the above may be true. However, many painful stories regarding health insurance surround breast cancer.

"Roughly one in four cancer survivors is unable to obtain adequate health insurance. It is not uncommon for an insurance company to double premiums once it learns that a subscriber has a cancer history. Insurance companies construct barriers to health insurance by rejecting new applications, canceling policies, reducing benefits, increasing premiums, requiring long waiting periods before pre-existing conditions are covered by the insurance, and excluding coverage for certain pre-existing conditions."(2)

The following helpful tips are taken from the sources listed below:

1) *Become insurance-literate*—or if it is too confusing, find a family member who will take charge. It's better if only one person is handling the insurance issues. Keep a log of checks paid and received and calls made and received. Write down dates and the names of the people talked to. Keep copies of all information you receive from your insurer. Don't throw *anything* away.

2) *Be sure you have read your health insurance policy completely and know what is covered and what isn't.* Highlight them with a colored pen, if that makes it easier to understand. Where areas are unclear, call the company. Find one person at the insurance company and always talk to that one person. Some policies require preapproval or second opinions. If you do not follow their rules, you may find you are loopholed in the future.

3) *Ask the insurance company if they have an 800 (toll-free) number.*

4) *Get all agreements with your insurance company in writing.* Phone agreements are not sufficient.

5) *Be sure that your premiums are up to date and that if you are in the hospital, someone is taking care of the monthly payment.*

6) *Be aware that "experimental treatment" may have different meanings in the insurance companies than in the medical field.* Insurance companies and Medicare often refuse to pay for chemotherapy that is used in a way not listed on the package insert, so they probably will reject claims for treatments the FDA has approved only for investigational, and not general use. However, if your insurance company refuses to pay for a claim for a treatment approved by the FDA for general use, appeal the company's decision. If you participate in an experimental trial to test a cancer drug, find out if the pharmaceutical manufacturer will pay for the treatment. In any event, if your doctor feels the treatment is justified, have him/her write a letter explaining why it is justified in your case, attaching medical articles, if any, that support the treatment.

7) *If the insurance company is slow to pay, contact your group representative at your office.* If you are self-employed, write a letter indicating you have sent a letter to the state insurance board and that the next letter will be to an attorney.

8) *If you continue to have problems, contact your state's insurance office.* Again, find one person who will help you—this is the only way to get bureaucracy working for you.

9) *Consult a lawyer for legal assistance if you feel you are being reated unfairly.* Sometimes just a letter from lawyer will make a difference.

10) *Get an answering machine with a call-taping feature. Just be sure to say that you are taping the conversation.*

11) *Consult with the hospital social worker if you are concerned about your health insurance coverage.* These professionals are often very knowledgeable and can refer you to specialists in the field of health insurance or give you advice themselves.

12) *If you are employed at the time of your illness, and covered by your employer's insurance, it probably makes sense to stay at your job, at least for the time you are receiving treatment.*

13) *If you leave your job, be sure to continue your insurance coverage under COBRA,* the Consolidated Omnibus Budget Reconciliation Act. This permits employees of large companies to maintain group insurance privately after they have left a job. It's expensive.

14) *If you are uninsured or have financial concerns, talk to the hospital billing department and your physician.* They may be willing to make special fee arrangements or find an appropriate referral. For information on low-cost treatment, call the American Cancer Society at 1-800-ACS-2345.

NOTE: *Due to major changes occurring in health insurance across the United States, be especially aware of your specific insurance policy changes. If you have questions, call your insurance company to be sure what the changes mean.*

Call the National Insurance Consumer Helpline for additional information on health insurance coverage: 1-800-942-4242.

Sources: (1) *Breast Cancer,* by Yashar Hirshaut, M.D., F.A.C.P. and Peter I. Pressman, M.D., F.A.C.S.; (2) *Charting the Journey,* edited by Fitzhugh Mullan, M.D., Barbara Hoffman, J.D., and the editors of Consumer Reports Books; (3) *The Breast Cancer Companion,* by Kathy LaTour; (4) *The Breast Cancer Handbook,* by Joan Swirsky and Barbara Balaban.

HOSPICE

"Hospice is a concept of total support and care for patients who have been diagnosed with an illness which will result in a limited life expectancy."(1)

A nationwide network of medical facilities, hospices are set up to provide supportive medical and psycho-social services for the dying patient, and loved ones. Usually connected to a local hospital facility, it has come to be one of the most valued resources for seriously ill patients with an estimated time of survival of about six months, and their families. Insurances normally support the cost, which is a set figure per day. The philosophy is to help make the patient as comfortable as possible, and assist the patient and loved ones in dealing with the dying process as a natural part of life, rather than making medical choices to save her/his life.

"People think a hospice would be a depressing place to work. It is just the opposite. I learn so much about about living, and what is important, from the patients and their families."
— Hospice Staff Member

Call the American Cancer Society (800-ACS-2345)
for a list of hospices in your area.

Sources: (1) "Evergreen Hospice Fact Sheet," Evergreen Hospital Medical Center, Kirkland, WA; (2) *Everyone's Guide to Cancer Therapy,* by Malin Dollinger, M.D., Ernest H. Rosenbaum, M.D. and Greg Cable; (3) *The Breast Cancer Companion,* by Kathy LaTour; (4) *Understanding the Final Messages of the Dying,* by Maggie Callanan Pflaum, R.N., and Patricia Kelley, R.N., *Nursing,* June 1986.

LIFE AFTER CANCER

There is a misconception that once a person has dealt with cancer and survived, that it is over. In some ways, that is the case. The medical appointments, the tests, the chemo bags, surgery, and radiation is done. But what has happened while going through treatment is that our lives have changed, and our perspectives with it. *Feistiness, an off-the-wall sense of humor,* and *a keen sense of what is really important to that individual* are a few of the "jewels" one emerges with from breast cancer. Every one of us would probably rather have gathered those other places.

There are some things that remain for a while. *Long-term side effects from treatment—physical, mental, emotional, psychological,* and *spiritual memories.* Some might be quite devastating, such as the loss of a breast, the restructuring of one's self image, or long-term chemical or radiation side effects from the treatment.

There might be *job changes,* or *loss of advancements, income* or *insurance* due to cancer. The best book I have found available on the many issues a cancer survivor faces is *Cancervive,* by Susan Nessim and Judith Ellis. This was partially written by a cancer survivor who eventually died, but was adamant about setting up a national support system for cancer survivors to address these important issues.

For the many practical resources available for the cancer survivor, read *Charting the Journey,* by Mullan, Hoffman and the editors of Consumer Reports Books.

The National Coalition for Cancer Survivors (NCCS), located in Silver Springs, Maryland, is a politically active national coalition of individual cancer survivors, health professionals, institutions, and regional and national cancer organizations set up to address the specific issues of the cancer survivor. It also sponsors an annual conference for cancer survivors and health care professionals. Call 1-301-650-8868 for more information.

A Political Choice: American Cancer Society Breast Health 90-Second Network has been set up to help individuals respond to breast cancer and breast health issues on a legislative and public policy basis. For more information, call 1-800-ACS-2345.

Sources: (1) *Cancervive,* by Susan Nessim and Judith Ellis; (2) *Charting the Journey, An Almanac of Practical Resources for Cancer Survivors,* edited by Fitzhugh Mullan, M.D., Barbara Hoffman, J.D., and the Editors of Consumer Reports Books.

GLOSSARY

Adjuvant Treatment: Medical treatment for breast cancer given following surgery or radiation to prevent any further growth of cancer in the body, either at the primary site or elsewhere in the body.

Alopecia: Partial or complete hair loss.

Aneuploid: Cancer cells that do not contain the standard number of chromosomes.

Autologous Bone Marrow Transplant: Removal of a patient's own tissue, which is stored and later returned to the same patient's body after chemotherapy.

Axillary Lymph Nodes: Lymph nodes in the armpit.

Benign: Not cancerous.

Biopsy: The surgical removal of a small amount of body tissue so that it can be studied under a microscope.

Blood Count: The results of an examination of a blood specimen in which the white blood cells, red blood cells, and platelets are counted to determine the balance and number of these elements in the blood.

Bone Marrow: The soft, fatty substance filling the cavities of bones where blood cells are made.

Breast Reconstruction: Surgery performed to recreate the breast mound, as well as the areola and nipple, following a mastectomy. A choice is sometimes offered to the patient to have it done at the same time as the mastectomy, or, more frequently, at a later date, often within a year or two. Some reconstructions are performed years after the original surgery.

BSE (Breast Self Examination): A woman's inspection and palpation of her own breast tissue as a preventive health measure.

Calcification: *See* Microcalcification.

Cancer: A general term for over one hundred diseases in which abnormal cells grow uncontrollably and invade normal cells. They then metastasize, or spread, to other parts of the body.

Carcinogen: Any substance that causes cancer or promotes its growth. For instance, tobacco, asbestos, and some pesticides (such as DDT) are all known carcinogens.

Carcinoma: A cancer that develops in the covering or lining tissues of body organs.

Carcinoma In Situ: The earliest stage of cancer, before the tumor has spread or grown significantly, and is still confined to the local area.

Chemotherapy: The treatment of disease by chemical drugs. Used before or after surgery, often in combination with radiation treatments. For breast cancer treatment, some of the more common chemotherapy drugs used are Cytoxan, 5-Fluorouracil (5-FU), Adriamycin, and Methotrexate.

Combination Chemotherapy: Treatment with the use of two or more chemicals to achieve the most effective curative result. Examples of combinations used for breast cancer treatment are: CMF (Cytoxan + methotrexate + 5-Fluorouracil (5-FU)) with or without VP (vincristine + prednisone), and CAF (Cytoxan + Adriamycin + 5-FU).

Cyst: An abnormal, sac-like structure that contains liquid or semi-solid material. It may be benign or malignant.

Diagnosis: The process of identifying a disease by its characteristic signs, symptoms, and laboratory findings.

Excisional Biopsy: Removal of a suspicious lump during an open surgical biopsy.

Genes: An inherited characteristic composed of DNA.

Grading: A description or classification of a cancerous cell or tumor according to its appearance and growth. Grade I malignancies are more differentiated, the most favorable diagnosis; Grade IV the least differentiated, the less favorable diagnosis.

HER-2neu Oncogene: A specific rapid-growth gene found in 30% of breast cancer.

Hickman Catheter: An intravenous tubing which is surgically inserted into a large vein near the heart, the end of which is tunneled under the skin and pulled out of an opening in the chest, then covered with a removable rubber cap. Medications, fluids, or blood products are inserted through the tubing. The catheter is used to prevent smaller veins from collapsing due to the repeated insertions of medications. Regular flushings with heparin, an anticoagulant, is done to prevent blood clots from forming.

Hormone: A chemical substance produced by glands in the body that affects other tissues in the body.

Hormone Therapy: Treatment of cancer by removing, adding, or blocking hormones.

Hospice: A program of caring for patients who are dying and the people who support them, with a focus on improving the quality of life.

Hyperplasia, Atypical: Abnormal cell growth.

Imagery: Visualization or use of mental images that come to conscious awareness in a deeply relaxed state to motivate the body's healing.

Immune System: The body's defense system.

Immunotherapy: Therapy that triggers the body's own defense system to control or kill cancer cells.

Incisional Biopsy: Removal of a section of a suspicious lump during an open surgical biopsy. The section is then sent to a laboratory for analysis.

Infiltrating Cancer: *See* Invasive Cancer.

Initiators: Substances or factors that cause direct cell damage leading to cancer.

In Situ: Cancer confined to the state of origin. *See* Carcinoma In Situ.

Interferon: A natural chemical made by the body to help fight infections, used in immunotherapy.

Intraductal: Contained within a duct. Describing a process.

Intravenous (IV): The infusion of drugs or fluids through the veins.

Invasive Cancer (Infiltrating Cancer): Cancer cells that have penetrated surrounding normal tissue.

Lats Flap (Latissimus Dorsi Flap): A breast reconstruction procedure in which skin and a piece of muscle from below the shoulder blade area are tunneled under the skin to help form a new breast mound.

Linear Accelerator: An X-ray machine that delivers external radiation therapy, commonly used for radiation treatment of breast cancer.

Lobular: Having to do with the lobules of the breast.

Lobular Carcinoma In Situ: Abnormal cells within the lobule that don't form lumps. Can serve as a marker of future cancer risks.

Lobules: Parts of the breast capable of making milk.

Localized: A cancer confined to the site of origin without evidence of spread.

Lumpectomy: The removal of a cancerous breast lump without the removal of the entire breast, usually followed by several weeks of radiation treatment.

Lymphatic Vessels: Vessels that carry lymph (extracellular fluid); a fluid that transports lymphocytes, a type of white blood cell, proteins and fats) to and from lymph nodes.

Lymphedema: The swelling of an arm or leg caused by an obstructed lymphatic vessel. A possible side effect seen following surgical removal of the lymph nodes.

Lymph Nodes: Glands throughout the body that act as filters for foreign bacteria. These contain special white blood cells that can trap cancer cells.

Lymphocytes: White blood cells that produce antibodies to kill foreign organisms and cancer cells.

Malignant: Cancerous, as opposed to benign.

Mammogram: Low-dose X-rays used to screen and diagnose breast cancer.

Margins: The strip of apparently normal surrounding tissue removed with a cancer or biopsy specimen.

Markers (Tumor Markers): Chemicals in the blood that are produced by certain cancers.

Mastectomy: Surgical removal of the breast as a treatment for breast cancer.

Metastasis: Spread of cancer from one organ to another, usually through the bloodstream or lymphatic system.

Metastasize: To spread to a distant site.

Microcalcification (Calcification): Tiny calcium deposits found in breast tissue, sometimes signalling the presence of breast cancer. Usually detected only by mammogram.

Mitosis: The process of cell reproduction or division.

Modified Radical Mastectomy: The removal of an island of breast skin with nipple and areola, all the breast tissue, and some or all of the armpit lymph nodes, and occasionally the smaller of the two chest muscles, the pectoralis minor.

Mortality Rate: The rate at which people die as a result of a particular cause in given population.

MRI (Magnetic Resonance Imaging): A machine that makes an image of the body by making a magnetic field and radio waves.

Mutation: The process in which the cell changes.

NCI (National Cancer Institute): A highly regarded research center in Bethesda, Maryland, that conducts basic and clinical research on new cancer treatments and supervises clinical trials of new treatment throughout the United States.

Needle Biopsy: Removing tissue from a suspicious area by inserting a needle in a tumor.

Neoplasm: A new abnormal growth, either benign or malignant.

"Nocebo": The negative effects of a doctor's opinion. With a "placebo," a patient is given a dummy drug and the patient responds because the doctor has told him he will. With a "nocebo," a viable drug is given, but the patient does not respond because the doctor has signalled that the drug will not work.(— Deepak Chopra, *Quantum Healing)*

Nuclear Grade: An estimation of the seriousness of the cancer by its appearance under the microscope.

NSABP (National Surgical Adjuvant Breast/Bowel Project): A group of research and clinical physicians who have formed a large cooperative group to study new treatments.

Oncogenes: These tumor genes can transform the normal cells into malignant cells.

Oncologist: A physician who specializes in cancer therapy.

Oncology: The study of cancer.

Open Biopsy: A surgery to obtain tissue for examination under a microscope.

Palliative: A treatment to relieve symptoms but not cure the condition.

Palpation: An examination by feeling an area to detect abnormalities.

Pathologist: A physician who specializes in examining tissues under a microscope and diagnosing diseases.

PCA (Patient-Controlled Analgesia): Use of a preprogrammed intravenous pump that delivers a set dose of pain medicine when the patient pushes a button.

PDQ (Physician Data Query): A computer service provided by the National Cancer Institute which provides up-to-date medical information on current cancer treatment.

Placebo: A substance with no therapeutic value.

Platelet: A type of cell in the blood that helps it to clot.

Poorly Differentiated (Undifferentiated) Cells: Abnormal cells that lack specialization in function and structure, usually indicating rapidly growing cancer.

Port (Infusion, Port-A-Cath): A small disc with a soft center that is surgically placed just below the skin in the chest or abdomen, connected to tubing which is inserted in a large vein next to the heart. Drugs or fluids can be distributed directly into the port in the body without multiple punctures in the veins.

Primary Tumor: The site where the cancer originally began.

Progesterone: One of the female hormones that prepares for conceptions and performs other functions before and during pregnancy. Certain synthetic forms of the hormone are used in cancer treatment.

Progesterone Receptor (PR) Assay: A test that determines if the breast cancer in a particular patient is stimulated by progesterone.

Prognosis: Expected or probable outcome.

Promoters: Factors that encourage the development of cancer but do not initiate the process.

Prophylactic Subcutaneous Mastectomy: Removal of all breast tissue beneath the skin and nipple to prevent future breast cancer.

Prosthesis: An artificial replacement for an absent body part.

Protocol: A carefully designed and written cancer treatment plan.

Radiation-Absorbed Dose (RAD): Same as Centigray: One chest X-Ray equals one tenth of a RAD.

Radiation Oncologist, Radiotherapist: A physician who specializes in the use of radiation to treat cancer.

Radiation Therapy: The treatment of cancer using high-energy X-rays.

Radical Mastectomy (Halsted's): The removal of the entire breast along with underlying muscle and the lymph nodes of the armpit. The result is a significant disfigurement of the patient.

Radiologist: A doctor who specializes in imaging studies such as X-rays, CT scans, MRI, and ultrasounds.

Reach to Recovery: A program for breast cancer patients that matches the patient with another patient who has survived. Organized by American Cancer Society.

Recurrence: A return of cancer when it was thought to be gone.

Red Blood Cells: Cells in the blood that carry oxygen and take away carbon dioxide.

Regression: Cancer that has shrunk due to therapy. In a complete regression, all tumors disappear. In partial regression, some tumor remains.

Remission: Partial or complete disappearance of the detectable disease.

Second Opinion: Recommendation from a doctor other than the treating physician.

Side Effect: A secondary effect from the treatment.

Silicone: Synthetic material used in breast implants because of its flexibility and durability.

S-Phase Fraction (SPF): The percentage of cancer cells that are in a specific stage (the synthesis phase) of division in the cell cycle. A high SPF number means that the cells are dividing rapidly and the tumor is growing fast.

Staging: The determination of the extent of cancer growth, a very important factor in the design of a treatment protocol. Systems vary by the type of cancer, but generally follow these steps:

STAGE 0: In situ carcinoma, no node involvement and no metastasis.

STAGE I: Localized cancer, probably without lymph node involvement.

STAGE II: Local spread of cancer, possible lymph node involvement.

STAGE III: Cancer has spread into adjacent tissues, definite lymph node involvement.

STAGE IV: Cancer has metastasized.

Stereotactic Needle Biopsy: A procedure which uses a needle placed by computer to obtain a biopsy specimen of a breast change that shows only with mammography.

Stomatitis: A side effect of chemotherapy that inflames the lining of the mouth.

Systemic Treatment: Cancer therapy that treats the whole body, usually using drugs.

Tamoxifen: A hormone therapy commonly used in breast cancer patients.

Tamoxifen-Chemoprevention Trial: Clinical trial of tamoxifen in 16,000 apparently healthy women to test whether it is safe and effective in preventing or postponing breast cancer.

T-Cell: One of the two major types of lymphocytes that are a part of the body's immune system.

Terminal: A very limited life expectancy due to illness.

Tissue Expander: A breast implant that expands the chamber connected to a port. The chamber is slowly expanded with weekly injections of salt water through the skin to the port. This is used in breast reconstruction.

TNM Classification: A system to classify cancers by the size of the tumor (T), lymph node involvement (N), and distant metastasis (M), (spreading to other body sites of the cancer).

TRAM Flap (Transverse Rectus Abdominus Myocutaneous Flap): A technique for reconstructing the breast by tunneling abdominal muscle, skin, and fat under the skin to make a new breast mound.

Tumor: A swelling, lump, or mass of tissue which can be either benign or malignant.

Tumor Marker: A physical change in the body that is not cancer but often occurs in connection with cancer.

Undifferentiated Cells: *See* Poorly Differentiated Cells.

Well-Differentiated Cells: Cancer cells that look similar to normal cells from the same organ, usually a less-serious cancer.

SELECTED BIBLIOGRAPHY

Table of Contents

BOOKS

Basic Resources

Dollinger, Malin, M.D., Rosenbaum, Ernest H., M.D., and Cable, Greg; *Everyone's Guide To Cancer Therapy: How Cancer Is Diagnosed, Treated, and Managed Day to Day.* 1991. Andrews and McMeel, Kansas City, MO.

LaTour, Kathy; *The Breast Cancer Companion: From Diagnosis Through Treatment to Recovery: Everything You Need to Know for Every Step Along the Way.* 1993. William Morrow & Company, New York, NY.

Lerner, Michael, Ph.D.; *Choice in Cancer: Integrating the Best of Conventional and Alternative Approaches to Cancer.* 1993. Commonweal, P.O. Box 316, Bolinas, CA 94924. (415) 868-0970.

Hirshaut, Yashar, M.D., F.A.C.P., and Pressman, Peter I., M.D., F.A.C.S.; *Breast Cancer: The Complete Guide.* 1992. Bantam, New York, NY.

Love, Susan M., M.D.; *Dr. Susan Love's Breast Book.* 1990. Addison-Wesley, Reading, MA.

McGinn, Kerry A., R.N., and Haylock, Pamela J., R.N.; *Women's Cancers: How to Prevent Them, How to Treat Them, and How to Beat Them.* 1993. Hunter House, Alameda, CA.

Morra, Marion, and Potts, Eve, *Triumph: Getting Back to Normal When You Have Cancer.* 1990. Avon Books, New York, NY.

Mulan, Fitzhugh, M.D., and Hoffman, Barbara, J.D.; *Charting the Journey: An Almanac of Practical Resources for Cancer Survivors.* 1990. The National Coalition for Cancer Survivorship and Consumer Reports Books. Available through The National Coalition for Cancer Survivorship [NCCS], 1010 Wayne Ave., Silver Springs, MD 20910.

Rosenberg, Steve A., M.D., Ph.D., and Barry, John M.; *The Transformed Cell: Unlocking the Mysteries of Cancer.* 1992. G. P. Putnam's Sons, New York, NY.

Swirsky, Joan and Balaban, Barbara; *The Breast Cancer Handbook.* 1994. Harper Perennial, New York, NY.

Strategies To Fight Caner

Allen, Judy Edwards, Ph.D.; *The Five Stages of ~~Death and Dying~~ Getting Well.* 1992. LifeTime Publishing, Portland, OR.

Anderson, Greg; *The Cancer Conqueror: An Incredible Journey to Wellness.* 1992. Andrews and McMeel, Kansas City, MO.

Anderson, Greg; *Fifty Essential Things to Do When the Doctor Says It's Cancer.* 1993. Penguin Books, New York, NY.

Benjamin, Harold H., Ph.D.; *From Victim to Victor: The Wellness Community Guide to Fight for Recovery for Cancer Patients and Their Families.* 1987. Jeremy P. Tarcher, Los Angeles, CA.

Bridges, William; *Transitions: Making Sense of Life's Changes.* 1980. Addison-Wesley, Reading, MA.

Frahm, Anne E., and Frahm, David J.; *A Cancer Battle Plan: Six Strategies for Beating Cancer from a Recovered "Hopeless Case."* 1992. Piñon Press, Colorado Springs, CO.

LeShan, Lawrence, Ph.D.; *Cancer as a Turning Point: A Handbook for People with Cancer, Their Families, and Health Professionals.* 1989. Penguin Books USA, New York, NY.

Johnson, Judy, and Klein, Linda; *I Can Cope: Staying Healthy with Cancer.* 1988. DCI Publishing, Minneapolis, MN.

Spencer, Sabrina A., and Adam, John D.; *Life Changes: Growing Through Personal Transitions.* 1990. Impact Publishers, San Luis Obispo, CA.

Risk Factors

Baker, Nancy C.; *Relative Risk: Living with a Family History of Breast Cancer.* 1991. Penguin Books, New York, NY.

Bristol-Meyers; *Breast Cancer: Risks and Prognostic Factors, Implications for Patient Care.* 1992. Bristol-Meyers Squibb Company, Princeton, NJ.

Eades, Mary Dan, M.D.; *If It Runs in Your Family: Breast Cancer.* 1991. Bantam Books, New York, NY.

McGinn, Kerry A.; *The Informed Woman's Guide to Breast Health: Breast Changes That Are Not Cancer.* 1992. Bull Publishing Company, Palo Alto, CA.

Rinzler, Carol Ann.; *Estrogen and Breast Cancer: A Warning to Women.* 1993. Macmillan, New York, NY.

Doctor/Patient Relationships

Jones, J. Alfred, M.D., and Phillips, Gerald M.; *Communicating with Your Doctor: Rx for Good Medical Care.* 1988. Southern Illinois University Press, Carbondale, IL.

Nutrition

Bradley, Jane, and Nass, Susan; *Nutrition of the Cancer Patient: Knowing the Major Food Groups Is Not Enough.* 1988. Nutritional Research Consultants, Dallas, TX.

Quillin, Patrick, Ph.D., R.D.; *Beating Cancer with Nutrition: Clinically Proven and Easy-to-Follow Strategies to Dramatically Improve Your Quality and Quantity of Life and Chances for a Complete Remission.* 1994. The Nutrition Times Press, Tulsa, OK.

Ramstack, Janet L., Dr. P.H. and Rosenbaum, Ernest H., M.D.; *Nutrition for the Chemotherapy Patient.* 1990. Bull Publishing Company, Palo Alto, CA.

Chemotherapy and Radiation

Bruning, Nancy; *Coping with Chemotherapy.* 1993. Ballantine Books, New York, NY.

Dodd, Marilyn J., R.N., Ph.D.; *Managing the Side Effects of Chemotherapy and Radiation.* 1987. Prentice-Hall, New York, NY.

Reich, Paul R., M.D.; *The Facts About Chemotherapy: The Essential Guide for Cancer Patients and Their Families.* 1991. Consumer Reports Books, Mount Vernon, NY.

Reconstruction

Bruning, Nancy; *Breast Implants: Everything You Need to Know.* 1992. Hunter House, Alameda, CA.

Bone Marrow Transplants

Stewart, Susan K.; *Bone Marrow Transplants: A Book of Basics for Patients.* 1992. BMT Newsletter, Highway Park, IL.

Shaffer, Marianne L., R.N.; *Bone Marrow Transplants: A Guide for Cancer Patients and Their Families.* 1994. Taylor Publishing Company, Dallas, TX.

Personal Journeys with Cancer/Breast Cancer

Bombeck, Erma; *I Want to Grow Hair, I Want to Grow Up, I Want to Go to Boise: Children Surviving Cancer.* 1989. Harper & Row, New York, NY.

Bulter, Sandra, and Rosenblum, Barbara; *Cancer in Two Voices.* 1991. Spinsters Book Company, San Francisco, CA.

Dackman, Linda; *Up Front: Sex and the Post-Mastectomy Woman.* 1990. Viking-Penguin, New York, NY.

Kahane, Deborah Hubler, M.S.W.; *No Less a Woman: Ten Women Shatter the Myths About Breast Cancer.* 1990. Simon and Schuster, New York, NY.

Kaye, Ronnie; *Spinning Straw into Gold: Your Emotional Recovery from Breast Cancer.* 1991. Simon and Schuster, New York, NY.

Ireland, Jill; *Life Wish: The Dramatic True Story of One Woman Who Fought a Courageous Personal War Against Cancer.* 1987. Love Books, New York, NY.

Mayer, Musa; *Examining Myself.* 1993. Faber and Faber, Boston, MA.

Pepper, Curtis Bill; *We the Victors: The Inspiring Stories of People Who Conquered Cancer and How They Did It.* 1984. Doubleday and Company, Garden City, NY.

Radner, Gilda; *It's Always Something.* 1990. Avon Books, New York.

Rollin, Betty; *First, You Cry: The Courageous, Inspiring Story of One Woman's Personal Triumph Over Breast Cancer.* 1980. Harper Paperbacks, New York, NY.

Wadler, Joyce; *My Breast: One Woman's Cancer Story.* 1992. Addison-Wesley, Reading, MA.

How to Be There for a Breast Cancer Patient

Dass, Ram, and Gorman, Paul; *How Can I Help? Stories and Reflections on Service.* 1990. Alfred A. Knopf, New York, NY.

Harwell, Amy; *When Your Friend Gets Cancer: How You Can Help.* 1987. Harold Shaw Publishers, Wheaton, IL.

Murcia, Andy, and Stewart, Bob; *Man to Man: When the Woman You Love Has Breast Cancer.* (or same book, different title: *Helping the Woman You Love Recover from Breast Cancer)* 1989. St. Martin's Press, New York, NY.

Spiegel, David, M.D.; *Living Beyond Limits: New Hope and Help for Facing Life-Threatening Illness.* 1993. Time Books, New York, NY.

See Triumph, by Marion Morra and Eve Potts: an informative section on family and friends of cancer patients is included. ["Basic Resources" section of Bibliography]

Personal Relationships

Bly, Robert; *Iron John: A Book About Men.* 1992. Vintage Books, New York, NY.

Bridges, William; *Transitions: Making Sense of Life's Changes.* 1980. Addison-Wesley, Reading, MA.

Colgrove, Melba, Ph.D., Bloomfield, Harold H., M.D., and McWilliams, Peter; *How to Survive the Loss of a Love.* 1991. Prelude Press, Los Angeles, CA.

Curran, Dolores; *Stress and the Healthy Family.* 1985. HarperSan Francisco, New York, NY.

Duerk, Judith; *Circle of Stones: A Woman's Journey to Herself.* 1989. Lura Media, San Diego, CA.

Estés, Clarissa Pinkola, Ph.D.; *Women Who Run with the Wolves: Myths and Stories of the Wild Woman Archetype.* 1992. Ballantine Books, New York, NY.

Gilligan, Carol; *In a Different Voice: Psychological Theory and Women's Development.* 1993. Harvard University Press, Cambridge, MA.

Keen, Sam; *Fire in the Belly: On Being a Man.* 1992. Bantam Books, New York, NY.

Lerner, Harriet Goldhor, Ph.D.; *The Dance of Anger: A Woman's Guide to Changing the Patterns of Intimate Relationships.* 1985. Harper & Row, New York, NY.

Limon, Will; *Beginning Again: Beyond the End of Love; Meditations for Starting Over.* 1992. Harper Collins, New York, NY.

Rosenbaum, Edward E., M.D.; *The Doctor.* 1991. Ivy Books, New York, NY. (Also available in video)

Schaef, Anne Wilson; *Women's Reality: An Emerging Female System In A White Male Society.* 1992. HarperSan Francisco, New York, NY.

Steinem, Gloria; *Revolution from Within: A Book of Self-Esteem.* 1992. Little, Brown and Company, Boston, MA.

Williamson, Marianne; *A Woman's Worth.* 1993. Random House, New York, NY.

Healing Mind, Body, Spirit

Campbell, Joseph; *The Power of Myth.* 1988. Doubleday & Company, New York, NY.

Carlson, Richard, Ph.D., and Shield, Benjamin; *Healers on Healing.* 1989. Jeremy P. Tarcher, Los Angeles, CA.

Chopra, Deepak, M.D.; *Ageless Body, Timeless Mind: The Quantum Alternative to Growing Old.* 1993. Harmony Books, New York, NY.

Chopra, Deepak, M.D.; *Quantum Healing: Exploring the Frontiers of Mind/Body Medicine.* 1989. Bantam Books, New York, NY.

Chopra, Deepak, M.D.; *Unconditional Life: Discovering the Power to Fulfill Your Dreams.* 1991. Bantam Books, New York, NY.

Cousins, Norman; *Anatomy of an Illness.* 1979. Bantam Books, New York, NY.

Epstein, Gerald, M.D.; *Healing Visualizations: Creating Health Through Imagery.* 1989. Bantam Books, New York, NY.

Fumia, Molly; *Safe Passage: Words to Help the Grieving Hold Fast and Let Go.* 1992. Conari Press, Berkeley, CA.

Gawain, Shakti; *Creative Visualization: Use the Power of Your Imagination to Create What You Want in Your Life.* 1978. New World Library, San Rafael, CA.

Gawain, Shakti; *Living in the Light: A Guide to Personal and Planetary Transformation.* 1986. New World Library, San Rafael, CA.

Goleman, Daniel, Ph.D., and Gurin, Joe, eds; *Mind Body Medicine: How to Use Your Body for Better Health.* 1993. Consumer Reports Books, Yonkers, NY.

Hanh, Thich Nhat; *The Miracle of Mindfulness: A Manual on Meditation.* 1976. Beacon Press, Boston, MA.

Johnson, Sandy; *The Book of Elders: The Life Stories of Great American Indians.* 1994. Harper Collins, New York, NY.

Klein, Allen; *The Healing Power of Humor: Techniques for Getting Through Loss, Setbacks, Upsets, Disappointments, Difficulties, Trials, Tribulations, and All That Not-So-Funny Stuff.* 1989. Jeremy P. Tarcher/Perigree, New York, NY.

LeShan, Lawrence, Ph.D.; *How to Meditate.* 1974. Bantam Books, New York, NY.

Moore, Thomas; *Care of the Soul.* 1992. HarperPerennial, New York, NY.

Morse, Melvin, M.D.; *Transformed by the Light.* 1992. Ivy Books, New York, NY.

Moyers, Bill; *Healing and the Mind.* 1993. Doubleday & Company, Garden City, NY.

Peck, M. Scott, M.D.; *The Road Less Travelled: A New Psychology of Love, Traditional Values and Spiritual Growth.* 1978. Simon and Schuster, New York, NY.

Probstein, Bobbie; *Healing Now.* 1991. North Star Publications, Georgetown, MA.

Roberts, Elizabeth; *Earth Prayers From Around the World.* 1991. HarperSan Francisco, New York, NY.

Rossman, Martin L., M.D.; *Healing Yourself: A Step-by-Step Program for Better Health Through Imagery.* 1989. Pocket Books, New York, NY.

Satir, Virginia; *Meditations and Inspirations.* 1985. Celestial Arts. Berkeley, CA.

Siegel, Bernie S., M.D.; *Love, Medicine, and Miracles, Lessons About Self-Healing from a Surgeon's Experience with Exceptional Patients.* 1986. Harper & Row, New York, NY.

Siegel, Bernie S., M.D.; *Peace, Love and Healing: Bodymind Connection and the Path to Self-Healing; An Exploration.* 1989. Harper & Row, New York, NY.

Simonton, O. Carl, M.D., Mathews-Simonton, Stephanie, and Creighton, James L.; *Getting Well Again.* 1981. Bantam Books, New York, NY.

Star, Jonathan; *Two Suns Rising, A Collection of Sacred Writings.* 1991. Bantam Books, New York, NY.

Life—Death

Eadie, Betty J.; *Embraced by the Light.* 1992. Gold Leaf Press, Placerville, CA.

Kubler-Ross, Elizabeth; *Working It Through: An Elizabeth Kubler-Ross Workshop on Life, Death and Transition.* 1982. Collier Books, New York, NY.

Leimbach, Marti; *Dying Young.* 1991. Ivy Books, New York, NY.

Morse, Melvin, M.D.; *Closer to the Light: Learning from the Near-Death Experiences of Children: Amazing Revelations of What It Feels Like to Die.* 1990. Ivy Books, New York, NY.

Journaling

Baldwin, Christina; *One to One: Self-Understanding Through Journal Writing.* 1991. M. Evans and Company, New York, NY.

Jackson, Jacqueline; *Turn Not Pale, Beloved Snail: A Book About Writing Among Other Things.* 1974. Little, Brown and Company, Boston, MA.

Life After Cancer

Nessim, Susan, and Ellis, Judith; *Cancervive: The Challenge of LIfe After Cancer.* 1991. Houghton Mifflin Company, Boston, MA.

Fighting Overwhelming Odds

Angelou, Maya; *I Know Why the Caged Bird Sings.* 1971. Bantam Books, New York, NY.

Bach, Richard; *Jonathan Livingston Seagull.* 1970. The Macmillan Company, New York, NY.

Caldwell, Taylor; *Dear and Glorious Physician.* 1959. Bantam Books, New York, NY.

Davidson, Art; *Minus 148 Degrees.* 1969. Curtis Books, New York, NY.

Frankl, Viktor E.; *Man's Search for Meaning.* 1985. Washington Square Press, New York, NY.

Gallico, Paul; *Three Legends: The Snow Goose, The Small Miracle, and Ludmila.* 1968. Pocket Books, New York, NY.

Hayslip, Le Ly; *When Heaven and Earth Changed Places: A Vietnamese Woman's Journey from War to Peace.* 1990. Penguin Books USA, New York, NY.

Hemingway, Ernest; *The Old Man and the Sea.* 1952. Charles Scribner's Sons, New York, NY.

Morgan, Marlo; *Mutant Message Down Under.* MM Co., Lees Summit, MO.

Mowat, Farley; *Never Cry Wolf.* 1965. Dell, New York, NY.

Read, Piers Paul; *Alive: The Story of the Andes Survivors.* 1974. Avon Books, New York, NY.

Steger, Will, and Bowermaster, Jon; *Crossing Antarctica.* 1991. Dell, New York, NY.

Thayer, Helen; *Polar Dream.* 1993. Simon and Schuster, New York, NY.

Uris, Leon; *Trinity: A Novel of Ireland.* 1977. Bantam, New York, NY.

Valens, E. G.; *The Other Side of the Mountain.* 1975. Warner Books, New York, NY.

Delightful Breaks from Cancer

Brilliant, Ashleigh; *I May Not Be Totally Perfect, But Parts of Me Are Excellent, And Other Brilliant Thoughts.* 1987. Woodbridge Press, Santa Barbara, CA.

Carroll, Lewis; *Alice's Adventures in Wonderland.* 1983. Alfred A. Knopf, New York, NY.

De Saint-Exupery, Antoine; *The Little Prince.* Trans. by Katherine Woods. 1943. Harcourt, Brace & World, New York, NY.

Grahame, Kenneth; *The Wind in the Willows.* 1969. Dell, New York, NY.

Herriot, James; *Dog Stories.* 1986. St. Martin's Press. New York, NY.

L'Engle, Madeleine; *A Circle of Quiet: The Crosswicks' Journal, Book 1.* 1972. Harper & Row, San Francisco, CA.

Martz, Sandra Haldeman; *If I Had My Life to Live Over, I Would Pick More Daisies.* 1992. Papier-Mache Press, Watsonville, CA.

Milne, A. A.; *Winnie the Pooh.* 1926. E.P. Dutton & Co., New York, NY.

Tolkien, J. R. R.; *The Hobbit.* 1966. Ballantine Books, New York, NY.

Williams, Margery; *The Velveteen Rabbit.* 1975. Avon Books, New York, NY.

Winokur, Jon; *The Portable Curmudgeon.* 1987. New American Library, New York, NY.

ARTICLES

"Adjuvant Tamoxifen in Early Breast Cancer: Occurrence of New Primary Cancers." *Lancet*, January 21, 1989, pp.117-120.

"Alcohol and Breast Cancer." *The New England Journal of Medicine* 317(20): 1285-1289, Nov. 12, 1987.

Barinaga, Marcia. "Can Psychotherapy Delay Cancer Deaths?" *Science* 246, October 27, 1989. [*Discussion of David Spiegel's findings that psychotherapy lengthened by 1½ years the lives of women with metastatic breast cancer*]

Begley, Sharon. "Beyond Vitamins." *Newsweek* 123(17): 45-49, April 25, 1994. [*A discussion of the phytochemicals found in fruits and vegetables, and the research ongoing connecting them to cancer prevention.*]

Borgeson, Charlotte; Pardini, Lani; Pardini, Ronald S.; and Reitz, Ronald C. "Effects of Dietary Fish Oil on Human Mammary Carcinoma and on Lipid-Metabolizing Enzymes." *LIPIDS* 24(4): 290-295, 1989.

Brisson, Jacques; Verreault, Rene; Morrison, Alan S., et al. "Diet, Mammographic Features of Breast Tissue, and Breast Cancer Risk." *American Journal of Epidemiology* 130(1): 14-24, 1989.

"Breast Cancer Research and Programs: An Overview." *Cancer Facts* [National Cancer Institute], May 27, 1992, pp.1-8.

Carter, Louise. "The Estrogen Decision" *View* [Group Health Cooperative] 35(7): 22-32, November/December 1993.

"Chronic Disease Reports: Deaths from Breast Cancer among Women—United States, 1986." *MMWR: Morbidity and Mortality Weekly Report* [Centers for Disease Control] 38(33): 565-571, August 25, 1989.

Cowley, Geoffrey. "A Scare for Pill Users, Is There a Cancer Link?" *Newsweek,* January 16, 1989.

Cowley, Geoffrey. "A Vaccine for Breast Cancer?" *Newsweek,* November 1, 1993, p. 68.

Cowley, Geoffrey. "The Hunt for a Breast Cancer Gene." *Newsweek* Dec. 6, 1993, pp. 46-52. [*The exploration of the familial connection in breast cancer.*]

"Detecting Breast Cancer." *Cancer Facts* [National Cancer Institute], February 1992, pp.1-3.

Dowling, Claudia Glenn. "Fighting Back Against the Breast Cancer Epidemic." *Life,* May 1994, pp. 78-88.

Eddy, David M., M.D., PhD. "Screening for Breast Cancer, *Annals of Internal Medicine* 111(5): 389-399, September 1, 1989.

Farley, Thomas A., M.D. and Flannery, John T.,B.S. "Late-Stage Diagnosis of Breast Cancer in Women of Lower Socioeconomic Status: Public Health Implications." *American Journal of Public Health* 79(11): 1508-1512, November 1989.

Fisher, Bernard, M.D.; Costantino, Joseph, Dr. P.H., Redmond, Carol, Sc.D., et al. "Lumpectomy Compared with Lumpectomy and Radiation Therapy for the Treatment of Intraductal Breast Cancer." *The New England Journal of Medicine* 328(22): 1581-1594, June 3, 1993.

Haybittle, J.L.; Brinkley, D.; Houghton, J. et al. "Postoperative Radiotherapy and Late Mortality: Evidence from the Cancer Research Campaign Trial for Early Breast Cancer." *British Medical Journal* v. 270, 1989.

Henderson, I. Craig, M.D.; "Adjuvant Therapy for Breast Cancer." *The New England Journal of Medicine* 318(7): 443-444, February 18, 1988.

Henderson, I. Craig, M.D., and Canellos, George P., M.D. "Cancer of the Breast, The Past Decade: Second of Two Parts." *The New England Journal of Medicine* 302(2): 78-90, January 10, 1980.

Karmali, R. A. "n-3 Fatty Acids and Cancer" *Journal of Internal Medicine* 225: supplement. 1, 197-200, 1989. [*Findings: dietary fat has a positive correlation with cancers of the breast and colon, perhaps others.*]

Lauder, Evelyn. "*Self* Breast Cancer Report." *Self,* October 1991, pp.135-145. [*A series of articles offered updating the public with breast cancer information.*]

Levine, Mark N., M.D., M.Sc.; Gent, Michael, M.Sc.; Hirsh, Jack, M.D.; et al. "The Thrombogenic Effect of Anticancer Drug Therapy in Women with Stage II Breast Cancer." *The New England Journal of Medicine* 318(7): 404-407.

"Lifetime Probability of Breast Cancer in American Women." *Cancer Facts* [National Cancer Institute], September 1992, pp.1-2.

Love, Richard R. "Tamoxifen Therapy in Primary Breast Cancer: Biology, Efficacy, and Side Effects." *Journal of Clinical Oncology* 7(6): 803-815, June 1989.

Mansour, Edward G., M.D.; Gray, Robert, Ph.D.; et al. "Efficacy of Adjuvant Chemotherapy in High-Risk Node-Negative Breast Cancer: An Intergroup Study." *The New England Journal of Medicine* 320(8):485-490, February 23, 1989.

Nash, J. Madeleine. "Stopping Cancer in Its Tracks." *Time* 143(17): 54-61, April 25, 1994.

Newcomb, Polly A., Ph.D.; Storer, Barry E., Ph.Dd: Longnecker, Matthew P., M.D., et al. "Lactation and a Reduced Risk of Premenopausal Breast Cancer." *The New England Journal of Medicine* 330(2): 81-87, January 13, 1994.

"The Politics of Breast Cancer." [A group of articles, including "Breast Cancer Prevention: Diet vs. Drugs," by Susan Rennie; "The Diet That May Save Your Life," by the National Women's Health Network; "The Environmental Link to Breast Cancer," by Liane Clorfene-Casten; "The Nation With The Highest Death Rate Debates Prevention," by Carolyn Faulder; and, "The Facts About Mammography."] *Ms.* May/June 1993, pp. 37-59.

"Radiotherapy After Breast-Preserving Surgery in Women with Localized Cancer of the Breast." *The New England Journal of Medicine* 318(7), June 3, 1993.

Rose, David P. "Dietary Fiber and Breast Cancer." [Review] *Nutrition and Cancer* 13(1-2):1-8, 1990.

Weiss, Rick. "Breast Cancer." *American Health* 11(7): 49-57, September 1992.

"*Coping*'s Annual Breast Cancer Report." *Coping* 7(5):41-50, Sept./Oct. 1993.

"X-Rays Beat MRI in Breast Cancer Detection." *Medical World News,* January 25, 1988, p. 53.

PAMPHLETS

American Cancer Society (ACS)
Publications available free
Call 1-800-ACS-2345.

National Institute of Health (NIH)
Publications available free
Call 1-800-4-CANCER.

"Breast Cancer: Understanding Treatment Options." U.S. Department of Health and Human Services, National Institutes of Health #872675.

"Breast Reconstruction after Mastectomy." American Cancer Society.

"Breast Reconstruction: A Matter of Choice." National Institutes of Health #88-2151.

"Cancer, Your Job, Insurance, and the Law." American Cancer Society. #4585.

"Chemotherapy: What It Is, How It Helps." American Cancer Society.

"Finding a Lump in Your Breast. American Cancer Society." #4586. Spanish version, #4595 also available.

"Helping Children Understand: A Guide For a Parent with Cancer." American Cancer Society. #4650.

"It Helps to Have Friends When Mom or Dad Has Cancer." American Cancer Society. #4654.

"Questions and Answers about Breast Lumps." National Institutes of Health.

"Sexuality and Cancer—Women." American Cancer Society. #4657.

"Special Touch Participant's Guide." American Cancer Society.

"Talking with Your Child About Cancer." National Institutes of Health.

"Talking with the Cancer Patient." American Cancer Society. #4557.

"Talking with Your Doctor." American Cancer Society. #4638.

"What You Need to Know About Breast Cancer." National Institutes of Health.

"When Someone in Your Family Has Cancer." National Institutes of Health.

Plus many others...

TAPES

NOTE: *Many tapes are available through local hospital libraries and support groups, and public libraries with no charge. Be aware that tape styles vary significantly. Feel free to inquire.*

Exceptional Cancer Patients, Inc. (ECaP). ECaP is a non-profit organization founded in 1978 by Bernie Siegel, M.D. Free "Books and Tapes Catalog" also describes clinical and other support services for seriously ill patients and their loved ones. ECaP, 1302 Chapel Street, New Haven, CT 06511. "For everyone interested in healing, growth, and personal development"

Siegel, Bernie, M.D., *Fight for Your Life.*

Siegel, Bernie, M.D., and Florence, Jerry, *Meditations for Peace of Mind.*

Simonton, O. Carl, M.D., *Getting Well.*

Simonton, O. Carl, M.D., *The Healing Power of Laughter and Play.*

VIDEOS

Because We Care. ACS #4666.05 *and* #4666.04 [*Describes basic service and rehabilitation programs for cancer patients available through American Cancer Society.*]

Breast Cancer: An Overview. Includes booklet. Irene J. Karlsen-Thompson R.N., M.S.N., O.C.N. (Updated yearly) Oncology Resource Services, 24539 S.E. 45 St., Issaquah, WA 98027. Phone (206) 557-9576. [*A conversational-style, updated presentation on breast cancer, covering an introduction, risk factors, signs and symptoms, types of breast cancer diagnostic and prognostic tests, staging, treatment decisions, follow-up, and future trends.*] Package price for video plus booklet, $41.00; or separately: video $33.95; booklet, $9.70, plus tax.

COMMUNITY RESOURCES

American Cancer Society (ACS), Tower Place, 3340 Peachtree Road N.E., Atlanta, GA 30026; 800-ACS-2345. [*Offers general information on prevention, diagnosis, research, treatment, support, publications, and referrals to services available.*]

American College of Radiology, 18891 Preston White Drive, Reston, VA 22091. [*Provides names of certified radiologists for mammography in your local area.*]

American College of Surgeons, 55 East Erie Street, Chicago, IL 60611; 312-664-4050. [*Provides names of certified surgeons specializing in breast surgery by geographical areas.*]

American Society of Plastic and Reconstructive Surgeons, 444 East Algonquin Road, Arlington Heights, IL 60025; 312-228-9900. [*Written information as well as a list of certified physicians by geographical area.*]

CanSurmount, 800-ACS-2345—Sponsored by the American Cancer Society. [*Brings together survivors, family members, survivor volunteers, and health professionals to provide mutual support and education. Goal: to match the patient with a survivor with a similar diagnosis. Call for information.*]

Corporate Angel Network, Westchester County Airport Building 1, White Plains, NY 10604; 914-328-1313. [*Alleviates transportation costs of cancer patients needing airlifts to NCI-approved treatment centers aboard corporate aircraft on routine flights when seats are available.*]

Encore, YWCA of the United States, 726 Broadway, 5th Floor, New York, NY 10003; 212-614-2827. [*Offers postmastectomy support and rehabilitation groups, with water and exercise classes.*]

FDA (Food and Drug Administration) Breast Information Hotline, 800-532-4440. [*Answers consumer and professional questions about breast implants, and will assist in registering complaints.*]

I Can Cope, 800-ACS-2345. Sponsored by the American Cancer Society. [*Offers a series of eight classes for cancer patients and their families, addressing educational and psychological needs of people going through cancer. Call for information.*]

National Alliance of Breast Cancer Organizations (NABCO), 1180 Avenue of the Americas, 2nd Floor, New York, NY 10036. 212-719-0154. [*Supports cooperative efforts between organizations and individuals in the fight against cancer, and serves as a resource for persons with breast cancer and other breast diseases. Politically active in insurance reimbursements, funding priorities, and health legislation regarding breast cancer at all levels. Prefers written inquiries.*]

National Cancer Institute (NCI), Office of Cancer Communication, Building 31, Room 10A-18, Bethesda, MD 20892; 800-4-CANCER. [*Offers the most up-to-date and complete information on cancer prevention, diagnosis, treatment, and ongoing research, with free materials. PDQ (Physician Data Query) offered, which provides medical information regarding treatments, and ongoing clinical trials. Available to the medical community as well as the public.*]

Comprehensive Cancer Centers, 800-4-CANCER. [*Supported by NCI. List of centers available that investigate new methods of diagnosis and treatment of cancer, and provide new findings to cancer doctors.*]

National Coalition for Cancer Survivorship (NCCS), 1010 Wayne Avenue, Suite 300, Silver Springs, MD 20910. 301-585-2616. [*National coalition of cancer survivors, health professionals, institutions, and regional and national cancer organizations that serves as an information clearinghouse. Offers an annual conference dealing with survivorship issues, a newsletter, and political involvement in cancer issues.*]

National Hospice Organization Help Line, 1901 North Moore Street, Suite 901, Arlington, VA 22209. 800-658-8898. [*Offers assistance in finding a hospice in a local community, plus information on how to start a hospice.*]

National Insurance Consumer Helpline, 809-942-4242. [*Offers answers to questions regarding insurance for consumers.*]

National Lymphedema Network, 2211 Post Street, Suite 404, San Francisco, CA 94115. 800-541-3259. [*Offers information about the prevention and treatment of lymphedema, swelling which can be a complication of lymph-node surgery.*]

Reach to Recovery, 800-ACS-2345. Sponsored by the American Cancer Society . [*Provides emotional and rehabilitation support for those with breast cancer, with hospital visits, a kit with a temporary prosthesis, and tools to assist rehabilitation.*]

Well Spouse Foundation, 17456 Drayton Hall Way, San Diego, CA 92128. [*A support network for those who live with, or choose to support, a chronically-ill patient. Quarterly newsletter.*]

Y-Me Hotline, Y-Me National Organization for Breast Cancer Information and Support, Inc., 18220 Harwood Avenue, Homewood, IL 60430. 800-221-2141 or 708-799-8338. [*Provides a wide variety of support services for breast cancer patients, families, and support personnel.*]

INDEX

ORDER FORM

QTY	TITLE	PRICE	CANADA	TOTAL
	Stealing the Dragon's Fire *334 pages*	$19.95	$26.95	
	Breast Cancer Charts & Kit *Please send me information*	TBA	TBA	
			Subtotal	
			Shipping and handling (add $3.50 for one book, $2.00 for each additional book)	
			Sales tax (WA residents only, add $1.64)	
			Total Enclosed	

Telephone Orders:
Call 1-800-468-1994. Have your
VISA or Mastercard ready.

Fax Orders:
1-206-776-1664. Fill out order
blank and fax.

Mail Orders:
Wilson Publishing
P. O. Box 12634
Bothell, WA 98082-2634

Payment: Please Check One

❏ **Check**

❏ MasterCard

❏ *VISA*

Exp. Date:
_____ / _____

Card Number _____

Name on Card _____

NAME	_____
ADDRESS	_____
CITY	_____
STATE	_____ ZIP _____
DAYTIME PHONE	_____

If this is a library book, please photocopy this page.
Quantity discounts are available. For more information, call 206-486-4316.

Thank you for your order!
You may return any books
for a full refund if not satisfied.